KETOGENIC DIET

The Low Carb Guide For
Long-Term & Rapid Weight Loss

**+ 40 Keto Recipes With Images
& Bonus Meal Plan**

Table of Contents

INTRODUCTION

Welcome, and thank you so much for putting your trust in me by choosing my book to read as your ketogenic diet guide! This book is packed full of helpful tips to help you get started and includes delicious low-carb recipes to keep you on track. Now, there may be a number of reasons you are reading this book. Maybe you are looking to lose weight, have lost weight in the past, but just can't seem to keep it off in the long run, or maybe you just want to find a way to cut carbs and live a healthier life. No matter what the reason, this book will be your new go-to guide for a keto way of life.

If you're new to ketogenic dieting, this will be the perfect place for you to start. I encourage you to go through the book chapter by chapter to see how this diet works, how to make the most of it and if this is something you think could work for you. If you're a seasoned ketogenic dieter and are just looking for some new and exciting recipes to incorporate into your diet, feel free to jump straight to the recipe section. This book features forty mouth-watering keto recipes to help make keto taste absolutely delicious.

Again, I thank you for reading my book, and I am so excited for you to start your ketogenic diet journey with me here today!

Example Recipe

Usually, when you're previewing cookbooks on Amazon, you'll just see an introduction or guide instead of what the recipes look like. There is a popular saying, "you can look but cannot touch," and in this case, you can read without actually looking at the end result. We will give you the ingredients, step by step methods for making the dish, and what the final product should look like. So I'd like to show you an example of a recipe before we get into the Ketogenic Guide, you'll find it below.

These recipes are Ketogenic and have been developed to be:

- Low-carb – All recipes are all less than 10g net carbs per serving, so they are extremely healthy.

- Easy to follow – All recipes have step-by-step instructions with detailed nutritional information. The ingredients are easy to find and put together.

- Easy on the eyes – All recipes have Images included to give you a view into what the end results will be. Moreover, this will serve as a bit of motivation to getting you on the right track of eating healthy. The brain's visual system helps us absorb internally everything we see in the world, so every time you look at a picture of a recipe you are subconsciously starting on the ketogenic dieting path whether you know it or not! Additionally, low-carb food looks and tastes good too!

Turkey Lettuce Wrap

If your keto diet has you missing carbs, don't worry because this turkey lettuce wrap closely resembles the gluten loaded wraps you used to enjoy while packing in health benefits instead!

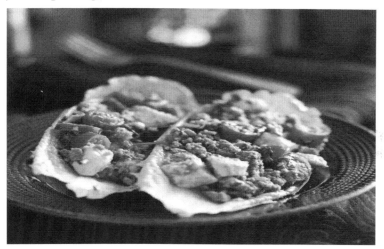

Dietary Label: (GF, DF, EF)
Serves: **4**
Prep Time: 15 minutes
Cook Time: 10 minutes

Ingredients:

- 1 lb. of organic ground turkey
- 1 tsp. ground cumin
- 1 tsp. garlic powder
- 1 cup of cherry tomatoes, sliced in half
- 1 cup cubed avocado
- ½ cup of fresh cilantro
- 8 large lettuce leaves for serving
- 1 Tbsp. coconut oil for cooking

Directions:

1. Start by preheating a large skillet over medium heat with the coconut oil. Add in the ground turkey and sauté for about 5-10 minutes or until thoroughly cooked through. Add the cumin, and garlic powder.

2. Next, add in the remaining ingredients, minus the lettuce leaves and gently stir.

3. Add two lettuce leaves per plate, and scoop the turkey mixture onto the lettuce leaf to form a lettuce wrap.

4. Enjoy two wraps per serving!

Serving Suggestions: Serve with a dollop of sour cream or unsweetened plain Greek yogurt for topping.

Substitutions:

- Swap out the cilantro for parsley if desired, and use grass-fed ground beef in place of the turkey if desired.

Nutritional Information:

Carbohydrates: 7g
Net Carbs: 3g
Sugar: 1g
Fiber: 4g
Fats: 11g
Protein: 27g
Calories: 226

HOW TO USE THIS BOOK

Part 1: Ketogenic Diet 101

Part 1 of this book is packed full of helpful information to give you everything you ever wanted to know about the ketogenic diet. I have broken down the basics and get straight to business teaching you the basics of this diet so that you can start your ketogenic diet safely, and have fun doing it. I will also talk about whom this diet suits best, and how you can reach ketosis, which is what everyone really wants to know! Use this section as your initial guide to navigating the ketogenic dieting waters, so that you can get started on your new way of life.

Part 2: The Easy Way to Get Started

Part 2 of this book is full of information on easy ways to get you started on your ketogenic dieting journey. We will discuss simple tips to help you get started, foods to avoid, foods to stock up on as well as the cutlery and gadgets that will make your life easier.

Part 3: Seamless Ketogenic Dieting

In Part 3, we get down to business and talk about how you can seamlessly start keto eating. We talk about the common ketogenic diet mistakes so that you don't have to worry about making them, as well as some tips on how to avoid those all too well know sugar cravings and how to stop them in their tracks.

Part 4: 7 Day Keto Meal Plan

In this section, I share a 7-day meal plan with recipes from the 40 mouthwatering recipe section of this book. Feel free to swap in any recipe you would like to custom design your own 7-day keto meal plan.

Part 5: 40 Mouthwatering Ketogenic Recipes

Throughout the recipe section of this book, you will notice labels and icons to make reading this book that much easier. The goal of this book is to provide you with straightforward and deliciously easy to read recipes so that you focus your time on making deliciously amazing dishes. You will notice the following labels on the recipes to help you determine if a recipe is suitable for your dietary needs and preferences.

GF: Gluten free
DF: Dairy free
V: Vegan
EF: Egg free
SF: Seafood based

Substitutions:

You will also see a substitution section below each recipe to make a recipe friendly for different dietary preferences. Each recipe will contain a dairy free and egg free substitution recommendation if appropriate for the recipe.

PART 1

KETOGENIC DIET 101

CHAPTER 1

WHAT THE KETOGENIC DIET IS AND HOW IT WORKS

"Nothing can bring you peace but yourself."

- Ralph Waldo Emerson

The above quote is one of the most important aspects of adopting a keto diet because only you can make the choice of what to eat. Only you will live this life and make the choices that will either help or hurt your body. Moreover, only you could create tranquility and peace in your life. Everything else is just external factors waiting for your responses. So, the simple question is what you are going to eat and which diets will you become involved with? There are many distractions in the world today involving food porn because of the tasty images floating everywhere from commercials to billboards, making you hungrier by the second. You need to have a strong will and never let yourself give in to the temptations because staying healthy and at an ideal weight is peaceful. Peaceful knowing that you do not have to deal with the pains and dissatisfaction anymore. This peaceful state could get achieved with a ketogenic diet.

If you're reading this book, you may be asking yourself what the ketogenic diet is? Many of us associate the ketogenic diet to be a low carb way of eating, but there is much more to it than that. It could be used to fight off diseases and help your body get into the habit of using fat for fuel instead of becoming lazy on carbohydrates. As a result, your appetite will get curbed and relieve any excessive eating habits. I can hear the "ahhs" already. Ultimately, your body will become a non-stop electrifying "fat-burning machine" running on an automatic weight loss regimen. Moreover, the visceral fat around the internal organs and excessive fat in the abdominal area will slender away with an associated uncomfortable inflammation feeling from time to time, but that indicates fat burning is occurring. Another benefit includes decreased triglycerides and increased good fat that will ultimately relieve high blood pressure.

We are going to dive into talking about what exactly this diet is, and how it works so that you can get started on your health journey as soon as possible! The path to weight loss is paved with many successes and benefits at the end of the road!

First and foremost, the ketogenic diet has been deemed a sure-fire way to lose weight. It has been used as a diet to assist in weight loss for quite some time now and is continuously gaining popularity. One reason for this popularity boom is that many people are noticing a rapid weight loss in only 10 days. The quick timeframe seemed surprising and unbelievable at the time to most people, causing them to research deeper into the claim. They could only find positive feedback from their friends, family, and strangers because the ketogenic diet served many benefits for many people. Those who engaged in the diet reported even treating epilepsy. Currently, there is more research getting done to really calculate the diet's effectiveness and how safe it is, which some doctors are in disagreement about. On one side, it is a dangerous diet fad that can have drastic results. In this case, always eating low carb foods can starve the body out of essential energy. On the flip side, the proven health benefits include lower blood pressure, decrease triglycerides and an increase in "good" cholesterol (HDL). Ketogenic dieting becomes a bit dangerous when people start using the Feeding Tube approach, without a qualified healthcare professional, by administering a feeding tube directly into their nose, down the esophagus and then exert liquefied food to replenish the body. Doing this could be quite dangerous; however, a natural switching in dieting is not. In 2016, ketogenic dieting was trending on Google for 14 months because there were so many people fascinated with the positive results. Moreover, new positive breakthroughs were discovered about the diet all the time, drawing conclusions that the pendulum is swinging toward the benefits. Ketogenic dieting is not like other diet fads that make unwarranted claims without following through. No, you could research the proven results. This 'unconventional' health field has world-class athletes and Navy Seals using it to enhance their mental and thinking abilities and physical performance. Consuming high amounts of carbs can cloud judgment and negatively affect thinking ability, making response time sluggish and the person lazy. However, low carb diets switch the brain into a more energetic mode that increases physical and mental performance.

What most people don't know, though, is that the ketogenic diet was discovered many, many years ago by a physician named, Dr. Russel Wilder of the Mayo Clinic. This diet has been around for over 92 years and was originally used as the sole treatment for those who suffered from chronic seizures. This was the only approach to treating epilepsy back in the 1920's before medications for this condition came on the market.

In the 1940's when anti-seizure medications came on the market, the ketogenic diet was not as readily used, and people lost interest; however, this diet sparked new interest as of recently, and more research continues to be done every day on the health promoting benefits. Many people are beginning to turn to this diet as a natural way to take control of their health as opposed to using pharmaceutical measures.

The basis of this diet is a focus on low-carb eating to allow your body to enter into a state of ketosis and a diet high in fats to keep your energy levels up and to help your body turn into a fat burning machine. The amazing thing about the ketogenic diet is that this diet does only assist those who are looking to lose weight, but research has shown that this diet is helpful in reducing symptoms associated with conditions such as Alzheimer's disease and is still used as a complementary measure to epilepsy treatments. There is certainly something to be said about this diet due to the science that has back its health promoting benefits for so many years and may be the hidden secret to reducing the obesity epidemic as well.

So, how does this diet work exactly? When you follow a ketogenic diet, you cut your carbs enough, so your body begins to burn fat for fuel instead of carbohydrates. This causes your body to go into a state of ketosis and allows for weight loss. Ketosis is a natural metabolic state helping your body burn fat for energy by raising the amount of ketones in it, which comes from a strict low-carb diet. For instance, when you are fasting you will notice an inflammation (burning sensation) in the belly area, which prompts most people to grab something to eat. When eating healthy, your body can regulate these feelings of ketosis by itself. As a word of advice, make sure to exercise during this process so that the skin does not hang, which is a major problem for overweight people who lose weight too quickly.

In the following chapters, we are going to speak in depth about how to reach ketosis and more about how this diet works. Head over to the next chapter to determine if the ketogenic diet is the right diet for you.

CHAPTER 2

IS THE KETOGENIC DIET FOR ME?

"The mind is everything. What you think you will become."

- Buddha

As with any diet, not all diets work for everyone and there are certain precautions that need to be taken before starting any new diet plan. Despite the fact that this diet has been shown to drastically assist people in their weight loss goals, and help with various other health conditions this does not mean that the diet is safe for everyone. The results of a bad diet can be drastic anywhere from strokes to hair loss, poor nutrition, premature aging, and even vitamin deficiencies. For example, I had a friend who decided to turn to vegetarianism in his early 20s as a result of studying about antibiotics and growth hormones that certain farmers inject into their animals to blow up the meat for larger profits. My friend was disgusted and afraid of this, so he decided to stop eating meat altogether. Additionally, he watched a documentary called "Meet Your Meat" on YouTube that sealed the deal. After turning to vegetarianism, he noticed that he had more energy, was better focused, and was happier; the world seemed different, like a permanent high. However, my friend started to slack up on his dieting plans and opted for cheaper processed foods such as Ramen noodles and pre-packaged meatless burgers. After some time, he noticed becoming light headed more, nutrient deficient, and eventually gained weight. My friend did not stick to the recommended daily amount of fruits and vegetables humans should consume for a healthy diet, and instead went for the large amounts of carbs, starches, sugar and salt.

To be sure that this diet is safe for you, speak with your physician before getting started. One of the reasons this diet may be deemed as unsafe for some is because they take prescription medications. There are a number of different medications in the market with side effects that may be impacted by starting a low carb diet like the keto diet. Certain medications may have a stronger effect on the body during the first few weeks of starting the diet, and certain side effects may be a sudden drop in blood pressure in those taking blood pressure prescription medications, and blood sugar levels may drop to a dangerous level in those taking insulin. The bottom line is always to speak with your doctor before starting this diet to make sure this is a safe option; they may request frequent follow-up visits during the first couple of months to make sure everything is within a safe limit.

Secondly, certain medical conditions warrant specific attention and concern before starting this diet. This diet may not be safe for those with gallbladder disease, or those who have had bariatric surgery. This diet is very high in fat that can cause the potential for issues for anyone suffering from either of those conditions. Those who are pregnant or breastfeeding may also not be candidates to start the ketogenic diet, as there is a high nutritional requirement for both mom and baby that the ketogenic diet would not be able to fulfill. The baby would need the extra amount of carbs for energy. A ketogenic diet can cause somewhat of an imbalance when the mother cares for another human being because the diet is mostly designed for weight loss. Some believe it is low in essential nutrients and vitamins that are absolutely vital for the baby to grow healthy. So, it is best not to take any chances with this dieting plan when breastfeeding. Another effect is a possible decrease in milk supply, which could cause dehydration and a lack of caloric intake for the baby. Lastly, those with pancreatic insufficiency, those who suffer from frequent kidney stones, or anyone who suffers from any eating disorder needs to discuss this diet with their doctor before starting. Eating disorders may be problematic because of the intense focus on food, and may not be appropriate. Always check with a doctor first because they will give the best advice for how to handle the possible health issues with ketogenic dieting.

The take home message here is that although the ketogenic diet has proven to have numerous health benefits and may be the answer to your weight loss goals as with any diet, it's critical to always check with your physical before starting. Your doctor will never steer you in the wrong direction because they truly know your body from the inside out. They have access to your medical history and will put expertise behind the advice they give. With any diet fad, it is important to do the extensive research yourself to get a general idea of the possible health concerns and then bring that information to your doctor and ask what they think. Not all diets are dangerous, but some could have their risks. If you check with your doctor and get the green light to start, you don't have to worry, and you can start the ketogenic diet without having to worry if this is something that is going to work for you. In this case, great, I hope you have great luck with the keto diet! Always veer on the safe side, your health is too important to take any risks. Cautious actions produce a healthy body.

CHAPTER 3

HOW TO ACHIEVE KETOSIS

"When the world says, "Give up," Hope whispers, "Try it one more time."

- Unknown

So, now that you know what the ketogenic diet is you likely want to know how exactly you achieve ketosis, and why you want to in the first place.

The first thing to address is ketones, and what they are. Ketone bodies are produced in the body when your body is metabolizing fats. When you are following a ketogenic diet, and your body enters into a state of ketosis, you will have an increase in the amount of ketone bodies in your blood which is evidence that your body is more efficiently burning fat. This is why everyone following a ketogenic diet wants to reach ketosis! A state of ketosis helps with weight loss.

So, how do you reach ketosis? Ketosis occurs when you deprive your body of carbohydrates by significantly restricting your carbohydrate intake. The ketogenic diet eliminates the majority of carbs and replaces them with foods high in fat with moderate amounts of protein. When you reduce the bulk of the carbohydrates from your diet, your body has to rely on fat for energy as opposed to glucose. When your body uses fat as fuel, the body begins to naturally burn fat on its own, which helps you lose that extra fat you don't want. So, the answer is that ketosis occurs when you restrict your carbohydrate intake and replace those foods with fats, and a moderate amount of protein. It's also important to not confuse ketosis with the ketosis that occurs with diabetes when the body does not have enough insulin. A ketogenic diet is an intentional approach to entering ketosis, and therefore this diet is dangerous for those who have diabetes since diabetic ketosis is already a risk factor. Type 1 diabetics often experience diabetic ketoacidosis, which has similar effects to ketosis. Healthy people practicing keto dieting do not need to worry about getting diabetes from keto dieting. However, they could develop Type 1 if they starve themselves for prolonged periods of time. This is why keto dieting requires that you specifically consume healthy food with low carbs so that a balance could be established. Not just doing a fast, which has its risk, but actually eating healthy food. Moreover, people with high blood pressure and those taking medications should not engage in this diet because of the risks involved.

You may be wondering how you actually reach ketosis. So, you know that you need to restrict your carbohydrate intake but what else do you need to know about achieving optimal ketosis? The first thing is that reaching this optimal state may take some time, patience, trial, and error. Most diets do not work the first time because everybody is different. You may need special attention to your body's natural biology that requires different approaches and some modifications. If you are an inactive person, who consumes lots of bread products, reaching a state of ketosis is more difficult than someone who eats healthy and goes to the gym. Don't lose hope if you don't reach ketosis your first try. This diet takes patience and adjustments to make it work. Stay knowledgeable about the different approaches in ketogenic dieting by reading online reviews from real people on websites like Amazon, YouTube, and blogs. Learn the adjustments they made to make this diet work specifically for them. The information is out there, and it provides great value to your keto journey.

To get started, you will first and foremost want to stick to a very low carbohydrate diet. Start by removing carb heavy items from your diet. This includes: bread, sugar, pasta, rice, potatoes crackers, candies, cereal (Yes, your favorite morning snack has to go!), cookies, jams, preserves, bagels, toast, pizza (We all love pizza, but it has to go, too!), sugary drinks, mangoes (Are you surprised?), sandwich wraps, French fries, sodas, muffins, pies, and sweet potatoes (this one is tricky because it is a great alternative to white potatoes, but still high in carbs).

Foods low in carbohydrates: eggs, beef, lamb, pork, jerky, fish and seafood, ground turkey, lean steak, veal, ham, salmon, tuna, chicken, organ meats, mushrooms, coconuts, garlic, raspberries, lettuce, cheeses, most vegetables, berries, and fruits.

You will also want to evaluate your protein intake since too much protein can throw your body out of ketosis as well. Foods high in protein: eggs, cottage cheese, swiss cheese, Greek yogurt, whey, steak ground beef, pork chops, chicken and turkey breast, yellowfin tuna, halibut, salmon, tilapia, navy beans, sardines, dried lentils, bacon, beef jerky, lean veal, seeds, nuts, oats, quinoa, and tofu. I know what you are thinking, all are delicious foods! Indeed, it is ok to eat these foods once in a while, but not too much to keep your body in ketosis.

Food low in protein: vegetable oil, cranberry juice, red wine vinegar, raisins, apples, grapes, mushrooms, noodles, macaroni, spaghetti, white and brown rice, orange and tomato juices, nuts, butter, cheese, bread, corn, any type of vegetable, sauces and condiments.

The first trick to reaching ketosis is actually to increase your fat intake! I know what you're thinking, increase your fat when you're trying to lose fat? Yes! You need to eat fat to lose fat, and you need to be comfortable with that concept right off the bat. Adding more fat to your diet will help to fill you up faster, keep you full longer and prevent overeating. Fat will also become your new primary source of energy, therefore it's important to eat enough of it. By eating adequate amounts of fat you provide your body and brain with the energy it needs to function, and it will be easier to enter a state of ketosis. Start by increasing food items such as coconut oil, ghee, avocados, and grass-fed butter. More healthy, high-fat foods include heavy coffee cream, whole milk, 4% butter, regular ice cream (Will give you the fat you need to keep hunger at bay), natural peanut butter, whole eggs, cheese, dark chocolate, wild fatty fish (salmon, mackerel, and herring), nuts, and full-fat yogurt.

You could integrate fat into your diet by cooking with it. This includes using butter and lard. You could also use vegetable oil, sesame oil, avocado oil, and coconut oil because they contain a nice amount of good fat. Another neat trick is to sprinkle small pieces of meats, squares of cheeses, different types of nuts, and dark chocolate on top of your meals. This is one of the reasons why most health-focused restaurants serve a variety of things sprinkled on their salads. They understand the minds of healthy people who are devoted to a specific diet. Moreover, you could add heavy cream to your coffee for that extra boost in fat. Eat guacamole in your spare time and even take cod liver oil in the mornings, then finish your meals with a nice glass of whole milk.

So, how do you know when you reach ketosis? In order to determine if you have reached a state of ketosis, you will need to measure the number of ketones in your body. There are a few different methods you can use, but the least expensive and most convenient is the home meter finger prick machine that you can pick up at your local pharmacy. To measure the number of ketones in your body, perform the finger stick first thing in the morning before breakfast. The number you are looking for, for optimal ketosis is 0.5-3 mmol/L. Anything higher than three mmol/L is an indication that you are not eating enough food to fuel your body, you do not want to get to this point. The key is to nourish your body with the right foods, not deprive it. Depriving your body will do much more damage than good.

Another easy way to determine if you've reached ketosis is through the breath test. If you notice a fruity smell or taste in your mouth, there is a good chance you are in ketosis. That "keto-breath" does tend to dissipate after a few weeks, so don't worry it's nothing long-term!

There are two methods you can use when first starting your ketogenic diet program. The first method is low to the high method. Start with a low level of new carbs per day, around 20 grams and once you start detecting ketosis, start adding in 5 grams of net carbs per week until you reach a low level of ketones. This is a very quick way to determine what your individual net carb level is.

Another approach to understanding how many carbs you need to reach ketosis is the high to the low method. In this method, you will start with a higher amount of net carb around 50 grams and then you keep reducing by 5 net carbs each week until you detect ketones. This is an easier method but may take a little more time.

As stated earlier, getting into a state of ketosis can be tricky when first starting out, and it may take some time for you to find the right balance. Don't get discouraged, keep trying. There are many fad diets constantly getting released into the mainstream that charge too much money for basic information, useless tools, and futile tricks and tactics. Some companies will mail you a basic health kit that includes a booklet, a pen, and a piece of paper and ask you to do everything on it that simply does not work. Some people will end up spending thousands of dollars on these new weight loss programs with no real success. Keto dieting is not like that. You make the choice of what you want to eat with no extra money is required.

A great way to ensure success with keto dieting is by keeping a daily journal about all your health-related activities, keep a separate journal about how you are feeling, what activities you are doing, and what you are thinking daily. Evaluating your mental processes and progresses, and making the right life choices shows where your mentality is at. Losing weight is mostly mental. If you do not have the willpower, then there is no way any weight loss program or regimen will have a lasting impact on you. Improving your mental and physical health will follow.

Jot down information about how much protein, carbohydrates, and fats you are consuming daily by getting a food nutrient servings chart or diagram. Read nutrition facts labels and take them into account every time you visit the grocery store or supermarket. There are many downloadable health apps that allow you to put in nutrition, protein, and calorie intake information and give results about your weight-loss progress. Moreover, documenting everything in the journal is permanent, so you could always look back at your past progress to see how far you have truly come, for more motivation. Create YouTube videos about your keto weight loss dieting progress so other people can see the effects of it. You will become one of those reviewers, I was discussing earlier in the book. If everything outlined in this book seems like too much work, then you could start with smaller goals before getting to the larger ones. Start slow and then speed up later. One way of doing this is by eating a few pieces of vegetables, fruits, and fish from time to time to get your body immune to healthy eating. Trying different healthy foods often will eventually lead you to some really tasty ones!

Do small exercises like running up the stairs, walking around the house, or walking around the neighborhood to get your blood pumping a bit and body immune to moving. This will prepare your body for the fat-burning sensations of ketosis. Moreover, when you are losing fat, you are essentially losing extra fat everywhere in your body, including the fat barring on your brain. This means that you will feel different in your outlook and personality a bit, however, if there are obvious warning signs of extreme light-headedness and internal pains, then consult a healthcare practitioner immediately. Remember, your life is not worth a diet.

Get help from supportive family members and friends for motivation, especially when the times get rough, because those unhealthy processed foods will eventually call your name, sooner or later, and you will need a net of people in your corner to help you stay strong. Stay focused on the road ahead and never steer off course, and always keep your family in the mind for motivation. Maybe get an accountability partner to help you with motivation as you both will push each other to success. When they start lacking in dieting and exercises, you could get them on the right track and vice versa. Keep reminding them of what you both are working towards.

Keep your metabolism going so when reaching a state ketosis, so your body becomes immune to rapid weight loss. Make sure your house stays stocked with whole foods and discard all unhealthy, processed ones. It will be very hard to let go of your favorite snack foods, but absolutely necessary for facilitating weight loss.

Take healthy snacks wherever you go and eat them whenever you have a taste for something sweet or get hungry. Only visit restaurants that are health-focused by looking at their menu options online beforehand to determine what they serve. You will need to toss the brochure of your favorite local chicken shack to the curb!

Never let go of your goals and stay mindful of everything you do. Change your mind about your feelings to ketosis dieting, and only associate ketosis with positivity. Change your heart by forgiving yourself for not practicing a bit of self-discipline and allowing unhealthy eating habits to take over. You are now a better person, so winning will become the norm. Stay in the winner's mindset.

Jumpstart your body by eating high-fat, low protein, and low carb foods, but always slide in a bit of each one to keep the balance.

This is just a bit of motivation to keep you on the right track.

Keep playing around with how many carbs you are eating, how much fat's in your diet, and if you are eating enough food for optimal body function. In the coming chapters, I will share a 7-day meal plan featuring the recipes from this book to help you better understand how to prepare your meals to reach ketosis, and remember to be patient and keep trying!

CHAPTER 4

WHAT'S A 'CHEAT DAY' AND DO I NEED IT?

"To keep the body in good health is a duty… otherwise, we shall not be able to keep our mind strong and clear."

- Buddha

Cheat days are something commonly found in nearly every diet program, to help you not feel deprived of all of your favorite foods as you try to lose weight. The question is, what exactly is a cheat day, and do you really need one on a ketogenic diet?

A cheat day on a standard fad diet is commonly an all out binge on things like pizza, cake, brownies, alcohol, ice cream; you name it. Anything you have been depriving yourself of is consumed on a standard cheat day. However, this is not the best idea with the ketogenic diet. All out cheat days can throw your body right out of ketosis.

Understand that you could still have a cheat day and achieve the ultimate weight loss results that you really want. A cheat day will bring sanity to your diet regimen because nobody wants to keep doing the same things forever, for the most part. The body will eventually come to a breaking point and scream out in agony because of those snack foods that you desperately want. Imagine chips and dip calling your name. Having a strong will is not enough because there is no amount of motivation that will overpower that snacking urge. The body and brain get fixated on having it. And this is ok. When feelings of depression, sadness, or emptiness take over, having a temporary food release will make a positive world of difference. There is nothing wrong with indulging in pleasure once in a while.

The concept of the "cheat day" was popularized in 2010 by the "4 Hour Body Guide" written by Timothy Ferriss. The main concept of the book is taking at least one day out of the week to enjoy your favorite snack food. Sticking to a strict diet plan can become somewhat boring at times. One side effect of having a cheat day is that you will notice food that normally gives you pleasure no longer tastes good. This is because your body has become immune to eating healthy

Let me share a personal story with you for a moment. I went on a fresh fruit and raw vegetable binge for about 2 months. I felt awesome. My outlook on life changed. And my positive attitude was contagious. Things that were normally annoying no longer affected me. I felt like a brand new person on an unexplainable natural high. Prior to this, I would sit and enjoy caramel sundaes and MCchicken sandwiches from McDonald's. That was my favorite meal and would do almost anything to have it. However, during my binge, I decided to revert back to some old ways and have a cheat day. So, I went to McDonald's and ordered my usual, getting ready for the pleasurable rush that I was about to get. When I finally bit into the sandwich and tasted the sundae after two whole months of not having any restaurant food, I wanted to throw up and spit it out. Surprisingly, my favorite meal did not even taste like food to me. It was bland and disgusting. The salt, sodium, and sugar were very strong, and I was disappointingly mesmerized. I actually put the order in the garbage. So, conclusively, the body can switch itself to crave a more natural diet, especially in the case of ketosis.

It is best to only eat the food on the cheat day that you love. This way, you will get the full pleasure and motivation to continue your ketosis diet. Chinese? No problem. Italian? Oh, yes. Whatever floats your boat. Make sure to eat small portions of it and enjoy the rest in moderation. Moreover, try not to pig out and stop when you feel full. Sometimes we have a habit of buying too much of our favorite food when we are really hungry!

If you feel like a cheat day, there are things you can do. A cheat day on a ketogenic diet is where you allow yourself an extra amount of carbs on a particular day. You would preferably want to choose slow releasing carbohydrates as opposed to processed and refined carbs. Some items that could be included on a cheat day would be things like sweet potatoes, beans, and nuts. It is also important to know that a cheat day is really only appropriate after you have been on the ketogenic diet for quite some time. Stick to the plan for 1-2 months before you start thinking about a cheat day, as cheat days if done wrong can throw your body out of a state of ketosis.

Do you really need a cheat day? If you can have a cheat day without going totally overboard, then you should be ok. Don't think about cheat days only in terms of carbohydrates either. Maybe you want to eat a little extra cheese with dinner, or amp up your calories for a day; this could be considered a cheat day as well. If you do decide to cheat with your diet choices and add in extra carbs into your diet, do so with slow releasing carbs and only have one cheat meal, don't make it a whole cheat day. Reaching optimal ketosis take a delicate balance and the last thing you want to do is to throw yourself out of ketosis because of your cheat day. After a couple of months of being in ketosis and you want to indulge, stick to one cheat meal and pick up where you left off the next day. Don't let that cheat meal turn into a vicious cycle.

Cheat meals are in place to serve as a way to allow yourself not to feel as deprived and to still enjoy things you really love, but they have to be done right, and they should not be done in your ketogenic diet infancy. Wait until you have some experience with ketosis before trying a cheat meal. Cheat your way to success!

PART 2

THE EASY WAY
TO GETTING STARTED

CHAPTER 5

TIPS TO SIMPLIFY YOUR KETO LIFE

"Peace comes from within. Do not seek it without."

- Buddha

Starting any new diet takes some times, and planning which is why I have created a list of tips to help simplify your keto life. Follow these tips to allow for a smooth transition into ketogenic diet living!

Tip #1: Avoid These Foods

- All grains - It is suggested to avoid all grains like bread, wheat, oats, corn, white potatoes, and quinoa because of the high carb content.

- Sugar - Sugar is one of those substances that literally wreak havoc on the body, and I will cover it more in depth later.

- Agave syrup - Agave syrup should be avoided like the plague because of the high sugar content. Actually, it is worse than sugar because of its low-level glycemic index. Agave syrup contains about 70% more fructose than corn syrup.

- Ice cream - It is ok to eat just a bit of natural ice cream to curb your hunger, but the main brands with lots of delicious goodies should be avoided. The best way to consume ice cream is to make your own.

- Cakes - Cakes, pastries, and cookies are high in sugar and should be avoided at all costs. Snack cakes are full of saturated fats, unnatural chemicals, and artificial coloring, offering no nutritional value. Most have unhealthy fats like trans fat in the shortening ingredients that will bring ketosis to a screeching halt.

- Sugary drinks - Check the Nutrition Facts on the back of sugary drinks and you would be surprised. Consuming sugary drinks during ketosis will trigger an insulin response which will cause a spike in blood sugar. Most "fruit" juices are basically Kool-Aid (flavored water with lots of sugar) in plastic bottles. The plastic itself is full of dangerous chemicals. There are plenty of low carbs, sugar-free drinks you can have the good. Sugary drinks will typically increase your cravings for more.

- Factory-farmed animal products and fish - Farmed raised fish is very dangerous to consume because they normally live in a very toxic environment. Farm raised Tilapia typically live in untreated pools filled with polluted water, living their life swimming in their own feces and that of other fish. Chickens are crowded together like sardines inside cages and basically live in their own feces. When they are finally processed, their meat contains so many bacteria that the handlers use chlorine to wash them off. Try to find out which farm your food is coming from and do research on how they treat animals. Avoid farmed raised fish altogether and buy wild raised fish instead. It might cost more but well worth the price for your health. Chickens, cows, and pigs get the worst treatment and when you watch videos like "Meet your Meat" you will come to understand why. When these meats are processed into hot dogs and bologna, they normally contain a nitrate chemical linked to cancer.

- All processed foods - Obviously, the difference between processed food and real food is that real food actually comes from real sources, but processed foods normally go through a machine and get chemically processed with all types of nasty chemicals and additives. Processed foods have chemically-refined ingredients and artificial substances that make them low in nutrients. Moreover, they are hyper-rewarding, so they are giving your taste buds an extra boost of pleasure that makes you want more. They contain every artificial ingredient from preservatives to colorants, making them a lot more addicting than regular foods. When you watch TV shows like "My 600 Pound Life" and take a look into some of the refrigerators and analyze what the cast eat, 9 times out 10, there is nothing else but processed foods. One interesting thing about processed foods is that the shelf life is usually very long, for years, because of the unnaturally dangerous preservatives that food companies add to them. Organic food typically spoils quickly because, of course, it comes from nature and when plucked from a tree or vine need to get consumed immediately because the fruit or vegetable will shrivel up and die. However, processed foods almost last forever, and as much as this sounds like a good thing, it is a bad sign for keto dieters. There are a couple of online videos showing how a McDonald's burger look after 5 years of being in the box and still looks the same from when it first purchased. Amazing. No mold, no nothing. This is because of the preservatives. When you consume those preservatives, they will preserve your body, not in a good way, but with sodium nitrate, sulfite, sodium benzoate that are all linked to heart disease, cancer, and obesity, just to name a few.

- Artificial sweeteners - Artificial synthetic sweeteners are very bad for your health because they operate like sugar in the body and are very low on the glycemic index. Some artificial sweeteners include stevia, monk fruit, and sugar alcohol. Some of the most popular artificial sweeteners include aspartame, saccharin, acesulfame k, and sucralose. Scientific evidence backs up the claim that artificial sweeteners are bad and can definitely kick you out of the state of ketosis.

- Refined fats and oils: Sunflower oil, safflower oil, cottonseed oil, canola oil, soybean oil, grapeseed oil, corn oil, trans fats. - Some of the refined oils to keep an eye out for are sunflower oil, safflower oil, cottonseed oil, canola oil, soybean oil, grapeseed oil, and corn oil because they all have trans fats. Trans fat is linked to horrific diseases because when they are heated, they oxidize and create free radicals which damage cells throughout the body. The majority of refined oils is genetically modified and partially hydrogenated, which are linked to heart disease and throw cholesterol levels off contributing to weight gain and stroke.

- Sweetened alcoholic beverages - It is advised not to consume alcoholic beverages at all because they will kick you out of ketosis.

- Tropical fruits: Pineapple, mango, banana, papaya - Although fruits are the best foods you can eat, tropical fruits convert into sugar once consumed. Anyone who suffers from diabetes knows not to eat tropical fruits just for that reason. Some associated effects on keto dieters include migraines, stomach pains, and most importantly would stall weight loss. Moreover, the heavy sugar content would make you crave for more snacks.

- Fruit juices - Surprisingly, fruit juices are full of carbs, artificial sugars, coloring and other harmful chemicals.

- Dried fruits - Most dried fruits are full of sugar and will throw your body out of ketosis.

- Soy products - People have mixed feelings about soy products; some say it causes cancer whereas others say it is completely healthy. It is best not to eat soy products and just stick with meats and fish for protein during ketosis.

Tip #2: Stock up on These Foods

- Grass-fed animal products - When animals eat grass they are producing natural hormones and energy that is good them and good for the environment. The meat gets processed into a superior quality because the animals are healthier and happier and has consumed natural foods from the earth. Unfortunately, most animal products found in grocery stores and fast food restaurants are fed growth hormone-laden food to make them bigger, so farmers can turn a larger profit. Many speculate this is one of the reasons you sometimes see teenagers growing up quickly because of the growth hormone laden meats they are eating.

- Wild caught fish - Wild fish comes from natural environments where they are eating bugs, plants, and other fish, but farmed raised fish are fed growth hormone-laden unnatural food to make them bigger for larger profits. Later we will cover the health risks of consuming farmed raised fish.

- Pasture raised eggs - Pasture raised eggs are the best for keto dieters and just people in general who are living a healthy way of life. There are many chickens that grow up in factories where they are treated horribly. They live in highly stressed situations that make them lose eggs, live under the feces of other chickens, and are not able to move. Pasture-raised chickens are healthier, happier, and produce eggs that taste better and are healthier.

Ultimately, consuming eggs from chickens with this type of energy will transfer to you and make you happy as well.

- Ghee - Ghee is an Indian and Pakistani version of butter that will give you a healthy dose of saturated fat. Moreover, it will boost the flavor of any dish you cook with. Mostly made from buffalo or cow's milk, it is nutritionally rich like coconut oil.

- Butter - Butter is a great low carb alternative for adding a healthy dose of saturated fat into your diet when cooking vegetables, fish, and meats. The beautiful thing about butter is the energy boost it gives you during ketosis. Maybe put a bit in your caffeine-free coffee in the morning to jumpstart the day.

- Coconut oil - Coconut oil is definitely the great white hope in the health community and is one of the most natural oils that you could cook your food in. It responds better and generally is healthier than saturated oils like canola oil and soybean oil and overall has a better taste. More importantly, it is low carbs and helps you burn fat. Some other benefits include fighting off infections and balancing cholesterol levels. Coconut oil contains medium-chain triglycerides (MCTs), which will help you enter ketosis easier by boosting the amount of ketones in the body.

- Avocado - Avocado is a keto-friendly vegetable that is very low in carbs and contains vitamin C, E, K all the B vitamins, zinc, iron, and magnesium. Avocado should be on your list of healthy foods to consume, and you could use them to create guacamole and sprinkle some cayenne pepper on top to enjoy keto friendly nachos. Avocados regulate hypertension and help lower blood pressure and perfect for a daily dose of fat.

- Macadamia Nuts - Macadamia Nuts are some of the healthiest foods in the world, containing omega 3 fatty acids, which helps increase focus, improve brain function, and promote better blood circulation, and palmitoleic acid, which reduces the body's ability to store fat. You can sprinkle them as a topping on your favorite dessert, such as brownies, or in a salad as a topping because of the monounsaturated fat they contain and flavonoids that turn into antioxidants in the body. Macadamia nuts are definitely power players in the health world.

31

- Olive oil - Olive oil is a very good source of monounsaturated fat that is healthy for the body. It typically burns quickly when heated because it is very delicate. Moreover, olive oil is a better choice for cooking because the body gets more energy by burning the saturated and monounsaturated fats better than the unsaturated fats found in their canola counterparts. There is no cholesterol in olive oil, and extra virgin olive oil is sweet enough to give you a jolt of energy and pleasure, while limiting fat and cholesterol.

- Leafy green vegetables - Leafy green vegetables are some of the most natural things you could integrate into your daily diet because they have many health benefits. Any kind of leafy green vegetable will be fine such as spinach, lettuce, kale, celery, asparagus, and bamboo shoots. Leafy green vegetables are some of the most nutritionally sound foods in the world that are low in carbs.

- Celery - Celery is one of the best vegetables for keto dieting because it has tremendous health benefits. However, some people think it tastes just too plain. So, if you want to spice things up a bit with celery, it is best to use some tasty low-carb ranch dressing, organic peanut butter, cream or blue cheese, or spinach dip with a bit of garlic sauce to really enhance the flavor. Celery has 0% fat, and one stick carries about 5 calories, so it is perfect for keto. A tasty alternative is to combine celery into a salad with apples, pecans, blue cheese, olive oil, and white vinegar.

- Asparagus - Asparagus is low in carbs and fat and is one of the tastiest combinations to mix with garlic sprinkled with a bit of sea salt to really bring out the flavor. Moreover, many people would cook asparagus stuffed with chicken Parmesan for a dose of high protein in their diet.

- Cucumbers - Cucumbers are very keto friendly. They could get added to a salad or drink.

- Summer Squash - Summer squash, also known as yellow squash, is very healthy sweet and healthy alternative to making stews and casseroles and grill with fish by adding some butter, sea salt, and Parmesan cheese. The food has properties found in it that will fight off cancer.

- Coffee - Although coffee does not have any carbs, caffeine could kick you out of ketosis.

- Tea: Black and herbal - Tea is a low-carb versatile liquid because you can add to it whatever you want. Maybe add some coconut, cinnamon, or even better to enhance the taste.

- Mustard - Finding the right type of mustard without any additives is very hard. Most big brand company's products are filled with sugar and salt, which would increase hypertension that causes high blood pressure. Some healthy alternatives are the Dijon mustard brand and whole grain mustard.

- Bone broth - For a healthy boost of protein to your meal, bone broth is the best choice because it is rich gelatine and minerals that will keep you warm during the winter months and replenish electrolytes inside your body to optimal levels. Beef marrow and bone broth are full of calcium, magnesium, and potassium, so they are very keto-friendly. They also increase the absorption rate of minerals. Moreover, they add good flavor to your soup.

- Spices - Believe it or not, there are several spices that have lots of carbs in them! You can use spices as toppings or taste enhancer. Cayenne pepper burns fat, cinnamon is low in carbs, promotes better blood circulation in the body, and fights off cravings. More great spices are chili powder, cumin, oregano, basil, cilantro, parsley, rosemary, thyme, garlic and ginger (boost metabolism).

- Mayonnaise - All mayonnaise brands are not created equally, as there are some better than others. Traditional mayonnaise is not a good addition to any of your recipes because the most popular store brands are full of refined, polyunsaturated oils like canola and soybean that causes inflammatory reactions in the body. Most brands have added sugar and salt to them. An alternative is creating your own mayonnaise from scratch or buying Hellman's or Kraft (made with olive oil) brands because they are health-friendly.

- Kimchi - Known as one of the world's healthiest food, Kimchi is a fermented Korean dish that should be on the menu of every keto dieter who wants to get a high dose of essential vitamins minerals. Kimchi is made with cabbage doused in fermented soybean paste and is very antioxidant rich, full of fiber, amino

33

acids, and most importantly low in calories. Astronauts eat this stuff in outer space to remain healthy and alert. Kimchi has been proven to aid in digestive health, fight obesity, and have anti-aging properties, regulate cholesterol, boost the immune system, and prevents stomach cancer.

- Sauerkraut - Made of fermented, pickled cabbage, sauerkraut is a good source of vitamin A, C, and K. It boosts energy and helps strengthen the immune system to fight off diseases. Moreover, sauerkraut promotes strong bone health and has some probiotic effects. It is a cultured food that also increases good bacteria in the body and will decrease the risk of cancer, asthma, metabolic condition, obesity, digestive and mood disorders, brain illnesses, and autoimmune diseases.

- Undenatured whey protein - Many bodybuilders use whey protein because it has awesome benefits. Whey is made up of the liquids that remain after cheese is processed and cured to produce a power protein substance. Undenatured whey is the best for keto dieting because it is not stripped of amino acids like biochemical processed, denatured whey. Whey is used to enhance muscle and build strength. A good way to consume whey is by mixing into a protein shake, sprinkle in a smoothie, or add to your ice cream recipe or milk when you need a brief boost of fat and protein. Whey is infamous for glutathione, which acts a quarterback regulating every antioxidant to make sure they perform at the peak levels.

Tip #3: Don't Deprive Yourself

Deprivation is a recipe for dieting disaster. Don't deprive yourself of calories. Your body needs calories to burn fat. Focus on high-quality fats, and a moderate amount of protein to nourish your body and promote energy. If you're hungry, eat! Just eat the right types of foods. Whip up a sliced avocado with a drizzle of olive oil, or make a piece of grilled chicken. Always eat when your body tells you it's hungry. This diet isn't about deprivation, so focus on the foods you can eat and foods like fats and protein that will keep you full longer.

Tip #4: Stay Hydrated

Hydration is critical for overall health. Be sure to start your day with at least 12 ounces of water, and stay hydrated throughout the day, your body needs it. It will give you an energy boost and keep you from becoming fatigued. A dehydrated body is a starving boy, so stay aware of how much you are consuming. One sign that you are not consuming enough water is if your urine turns yellow. Increase your fluid intake during exercise as well, and add a pinch of sea salt to your gym water bottle to replace essential electrolytes. Staying hydrated will promote proper digestion in the internal systems because your body craves more water when going through keto dieting. Also, drinking more water to help relieve the symptoms of "keto breath" (fruity or foul).

Tip #5: Consume Enough Sea Salt

When you follow a low-carb diet, your body needs a little extra sodium, from the right sources. Our kidneys excrete more sodium on a keto diet due to the lower insulin levels. Try adding a teaspoon of Himalayan sea salt into your diet daily, or try some sea veggies such as nori, or kelp to enjoy natural foods high in sodium

Tip #6: Beat Constipation

Constipation can be a huge issue for keto dieters. To remedy this problem consider magnesium supplementation based on doctors approval, and increase your probiotic rich foods such as kimchi, and sauerkraut. Staying hydrated will also help to keep the bowels moving. You could consume more fibrous vegetables and fermented foods to relieve the painful strain. Drink more electrolyte water to replace the sodium, potassium, and calcium used by your body to makes things flow smoothly. Avoid stressful situations that are causing more strain in your life because it could cause more strain in the bathroom.

Tip #7: Exercise Regularly

Exercise is an important part of a healthy lifestyle and can help you along your keto journey as well. Regular exercise with resistance training and exercise can help balance blood sugar levels and help you reach a state of ketosis.

Tip # 8: Fasting

Fasting is a very important way to get your body into a state of ketosis because you are essentially going without certain foods that you usually have a craving for. Going without food is a mild form of ketosis, and the best way to prepare for a keto diet is by intermittent fasting which includes skipping meals throughout the week. This will get your body into the rhythm of going without food. It will be difficult at first, but as time passes you will start to feel different about your food choices and develop a tolerance for going without food. Moreover, fasting before a keto diet will help you avoid a hypoglycemic event. So, in a sense, you are cleansing yourself in preparation to help maintain ketosis.

Tip #9: Test Ketone Levels

Testing your ketone level is essential to finding out if you are on the right track to ketosis. Visiting your local doctor and having them perform a ketone test or using a personal meter purchased from a drug store could help you test ketones properly. From there, you can make the proper adjustments. The three major ketones to look out for are acetone, beta-hydroxybutyrate, and acetoacetate. They are normally measured in blood, breath, and urine.

Follow these tips to help you seamlessly enter into a state of ketosis and start your weight loss journey without stress. This diet takes a little bit of planning, but with these steps, you will be well on your way to keto success.

CHAPTER 6

WHAT CUTLERY AND GADGETS WILL HELP?

*"As I see it, every day you do one of two things:
build health or produce disease in yourself."*

- Adelle Davis

Before you begin your ketogenic journey, it's important to plan what cutlery and gadgets may help make your life just that much easier! Prepping your kitchen for success is one of the key components of being successful in this diet. Here is some of the cutlery and gadgets that may help you reach ketosis, and make this diet simple and fun.

Cutlery:

- Blender - Although a smoothie is high in carbs, getting a blender will allow you to make choices about the ingredients. You could have a nice, healthy liquid concoction of your liking, especially if you want to stay away from solid foods. In fact, the body is able to absorb more vitamins and minerals from food in a liquid form than solid. Moreover, you could add a bit of natural ice cream and whole milk for a boost of fat or protein. After blending fruits and vegetables together into juice form, you could pour the mushy remainder into a Popsicle molder to create your own flavorful ice cream bar. One of the best types of blenders for making a nice ketogenic drink is the Magic Bullet. Take multivitamins along with your smoothie to fill you up for the day and keep your body in ketosis to becoming free of fat!

- Food processor - A food processor is a nifty tool that will automatically turn food into really small pieces, which is pretty fun to eat if you like a gritty taste. Grind cauliflower or broccoli like mashed potatoes and smother them with bone broth gravy. A hard block of cheese? No problem. Grind it and sprinkle on top of your favorite dish. Food processors chop, slice, or shred anything that stands in its way, making it a versatile tool if you have creative cooking ideas. Add your favorite keto-friendly ingredients all at once and pulse almonds into milk that is antibiotic and preservative free. Cuisinart has great food processors that you can buy at affordable prices.

- Skillet - The skillet will be used to cook up most of the recipes in this book with no problems. The best type of skillet to purchase is a cast iron one because it does not stick, allowing you to make anything from glazed salmon, low carb pizza, to brownies and even ice cream.

- Immersion blender - This would be a great tool to make your mashed potatoes and soups in. They would turn into a liquid less thick than what a blender does, depending on how long you leave food in there, perfect for merging fruits and veggies together. If you like a mashed potato texture, then blend some cauliflower for that genuine mash taste. Or, have some bone broth and soup blended together perfectly. An immersion blender could blend different types of soups, sauces, and liquids to create the perfect delectable combination.

- Slow-cooker - Using a slow-cooker have many benefits, and on a psychological level, it will test your patience. You need to sit around and wait for the food to get done, which is why some people get anxious and prefer the fast food option. A slow-cooker takes a concentrated effort to bring a nice meal together. Moreover, it will give you great confidence knowing that you have cooked from scratch. One of the best slow cooker brands is by Hamilton Beach.

- Veggie Spiralizer - A veggie spiralizer is definitely a fun way of making a dish more attractive and motivating to eat. Imagine stringy vegetables strewn on top of your favorite keto dish, bringing a new dynamic in the dining room. Fixing the dishes would take on a whole new meaning as you stir fry stringy vegetables in coconut oil sprinkled with a bit of sea salt. Instead of using starched and carb filled Ramen noodles that convert into extra sugar in your body, how about creating some beautifully crafted broccoli or zucchini noodles? They are healthy and taste better! Sometimes we attract to food by how it looks on the plate, which is why Michelin star restaurants focus on creating artisanal works of art, and the delicious tastes are just icing on the cake. After the recipes, you could simply add some stringy vegetables on top of a dish or as a complementary side. Parmesan chicken here we come!

- Veggie Chopper - This little gadget provides lots of fun that adds a different dynamic to the way you eat fruits and vegetables. You will be able to chop up fruits and vegetables into smaller pieces to combine into a salad or as a topping for your breakfast or lunch dishes. This would be the perfect way to get the proper daily servings of fruits and vegetables. Blend strawberries, blueberries, or raspberries together for a genuine berry blast or chop some pineapples, apples, bananas, and watermelon for a fruit fusion.

- Coffee Maker - It is very difficult to add those coffee additives for a taste of fat that you need, especially when the line at Starbucks during the rush hour traffic when everyone is waiting in life. Making coffee at home takes a concentrated effort, and most importantly, you can add whatever you want. That means no caffeine.

- Glass Tupperware storage containers - Glass Tupperware storage containers are best for storing food in the refrigerator for an extended period of time to keep it fresh. The glassed ones are better than plastic because they do not leach petrochemicals and xenoestrogens that are commonly found in plastics, essentially poisoning the food.

- Hand-held mixer - An essential tool found in almost every kitchen that takes food seriously are electric handheld mixer to liquefy your substances. Commonly used to beat up egg whites and whipping creams.

- Kitchen Knives - Kitchen knives come in different shapes, sizes, types, and sharpness. A word of advice: Always keep your blades sharp to cut into food more easily because a dull knife will make you put more pressure into cutting, which could slip and cause an injury. Simple kitchen knives are easier to work and store.

However, if you decide to buy some that are a bit complex then get some that are high-quality.

- Parchment paper - A durable, heat-resistant, non-stick paper that is easy to clean up and perfect for cooking fish, unlike aluminum and wax paper.

- Baking pans and sheets - These are the basic tools to cook the majority of the dishes in this book.

- Popsicle molds - After using the blender to create the mushy fruit-filled concoction, you can simply fuse it into the Popsicle molds sprinkled with just a bit of spirulina and wheatgrass and pop in the freezer.

- Measuring jugs - Following a specific keto recipe would be easier with a measuring jug to know the proper amounts of ingredients to add to a dish. Whether it is a breakfast or dinner dish, making you sure you have the right amount of butter, water, seasonings, and spices are essential. Too much of anything is bad and could mess up the dish. Sometimes it may come out too salty, too rich in flavor, or not have enough moisture.

- Lemon squeezer - Sometimes doing work around the house while on a keto diet could get tiring at times and one way for an energy boost is to use a fruit squeezer to create a natural juice. This will give a needed energy boost with the right amount of natural sugars to keep going. Squeeze your favorite lemons, oranges, and apples into a juice for that genuine flavorful fruity taste without the associated refined sugars commonly found in processed fruit juices (Kool-Aid).

- Ice cream maker - This little, sweet machine is perfect for making a healthy dessert for the lunches and dinner dishes, especially as a reward for a job well done. It is ok to reward yourself with a bit of ice cream for a healthy dose of fat, but when you are the master chef in the kitchen creating the ice cream yourself, then it is so much better. Moreover, you could give your personalized ice cream flavor a real health boost by adding spirulina wheatgrass, organic nuts, or any tasty, healthy alternatives with keto-friendly sweeteners on top.

- Smoking - Smoking your meat is a fun and tasty way to enjoy your keto diet. It will also test your patience as well. Enjoy a healthy dose of fat by cooking fresh and wild fish.

Gadgets:

- Ketone body tester: You get a finger prick machine from your local pharmacy. They are affordable and easy to use, similar to a diabetic machine. They perform a "spot test," in which the blood is dipped and the chemical reacts to the ketones. There is also a urine test that gets performed at the doctor.

- Pedometer or fitness tracker if you plan to track your exercise.

PART 3

SEAMLESS KETO DIETING

CHAPTER 7

COMMON KETOGENIC MISTAKES

"Never mistake a single mistake with a final mistake."

- F. Scott Fitzgerald

Everyone makes dieting mistakes, especially when you may be unsure as to how to correctly follow the diet guidelines. This is why I have created a list of some of the top ketogenic dieting mistakes to help you prevent making them, and so you can seamlessly start your ketogenic diet.

#1: Eating too Many Carbs

This is more of an obvious one, but one that happens quite frequently when you start eating a ketogenic diet. This occurs more if you don't take the proper steps in determining what your optimal net carb intake is. Once you know that number, it's harder to overeat carbohydrates. Remember to measure the number of ketones in your body, and as a rough estimate, the number of carbs one should be eating is roughly 20-50 grams per day. However, everyone is different, so be sure to follow the low to high or the high to a low method to determine how many net carbs your body requires for ketosis. This will be a unique number that works specifically for you.

#2: Eating too Much Protein

Although the ketogenic diet is based on low-carb eating too much protein is not good either! When you eat more protein than your body requires, some of those extra amino acids will turn into glucose. This can throw your body out of ketosis, so don't go overdoing your post workout protein shakes! To be sure you aren't overeating in the protein department, try to stick with 0.7-0.9 grams of protein per pound of body weight and go for 0.9 grams of protein per pound if you are extremely active.

#3: Not Eating Enough Fat

This diet is only effective if you eat the proper amount of fat! Don't be afraid of fat, especially healthy sources such as coconut, olive, and grass fed butter. Your body needs this for energy, now that you are eliminating a large majority of carbohydrate sources. Don't restrict fats or you will be in for some major mood swings, you will constantly feel hungry, and your body will start to break down because it has nothing else to rely on for fuel. Don't damage your body by restricting fats.

#4: Not Being Patient

As we have previously talked about, many people throw in the towel too soon and think that this diet doesn't work. The truth is that ketogenic dieting takes some time, and it certainly takes patience! Play around with your carbohydrate intake, increase fats if needed, and don't be discouraged by those yucky symptoms you may experience the first couple of days starting this diet. Some people quit very early on because they may feel a little under the weather a few days after eliminating many of the carbs from their diet. Be mindful and patient with yourself in knowing that your body is going through a huge adjustment period and just needs time to adapt.

#5: You Are Not Fully Committed

Rome wasn't built in a day, and keto dieting will not become successful during this timeframe either. Let's say you have read all the information about ketogenic dieting and completed just some of the steps, but not all of them. This means you are not fully committed to your goals and are just testing out the methods for fun. Being halfway involved would not cut it because it takes a full committed effort for successful in this diet. Avoid all distractions and lock into keto dieting by exclusively focusing on that. It needs to become part of your life. If you only used half the energy to study at a university and get C's throughout the 4 years, eventually your grade point average would decrease, putting your entire education degree in jeopardy. To be successful, you need some to squeeze some A's and B's in there to boost your grade point average. Staying fully determined is the key to success with ketogenic dieting. Even when certain methods do not work, switch them or keep trying until they work.

#6: Watching The Scale Like A Hawk

With eagle eyes, you are becoming fixated on the scale like a hawk. There are some people who literally want to get on the scale after every workout just to see if there was some progress being made. Focusing on the scale would not do the trick, however, focusing on changing lifestyle choices and changing your outlook on life would help improve the effects of keto dieting. This diet should become part of your daily activities. You should stay so engrossed with the plan that it becomes second nature, an effortlessly subconscious action. After a while, the scale should not matter anymore because you will feel skinny and mentally become skinny, and then the body will follow only if you are practicing the diet every day correctly. Only use the scale as motivation. Also, keep in mind that weight can fluctuate, depending on what you have eaten or drank the night before. Factor in what you have eaten for breakfast and what you are wearing, so the scale would read the true weight.

#7: Expecting A Quick Fix

Short term goals equal to short terms results and successes because anything worth having will require much work. This is repeated in so many ways throughout the years by so many philosophers and is truer now than ever before. Keto dieting is a long-term process because it requires you make near-permanent lifestyle changes and adopt responsible eating habits. Although you can lose a lot of weight in 10 days, which is the main draw of the keto diet, there is still plenty of work that needs to get done. Even people who decide to leap over all the obese people and land in the world of liposuction and tummy tucks, they still need to adhere to a strict diet for months or even years, so the weight stays off.

#8: Not Planning

Planning your keto diet ahead of time is essential to success in weight loss. So, it is best to do plenty of research with books like this one that could be found in the library, Amazon, or Barnes and Noble, look up health publications about keto dieting and read scientific journals to see what the scientists are saying. Access YouTube and read reviews about keto dieting and then make notes about what needs to get done for ketosis to take place. Just getting into a diet with no knowledge, preparation, or support is drastic and will prove to be futile in the end. Do not learn the important stuff along the way, but instead do research up front, so mistakes are avoided. Prepare in advance to execute with success. Stay ready, so you do not need to get ready.

#9. Not Getting An Accountability Partner

Getting someone to accompany you for the ride on your weight loss regimen will give you a sense of camaraderie, motivation, and accomplishment. Sometimes having friend who is on your side guiding you along the journey could spell the difference between success and disaster. We think we know it all and could do things ourselves, but sometimes we need someone watching our backs for help. This works especially well if you are the type of person who is an extrovert, outgoing person. Others can learn from you and lean on you for support during their keto dieting. There is nothing wrong with having someone keeping you on your feet. Get an accountability partner so you both can ride into the sunset together.

#10: Not Bringing Enough Balance To Your Life

People have a habit of focusing only on one thing at a time by zeroing in on it, which is great. This is how we stay focused on responsibilities and complete tasks on time. And staying focused is essential to keto dieting. However, you should always stay versatile in your approaches to keto dieting as well. Make sure the water you drink is vitamin water or electrolyte water, especially when doing rigorous workouts because you lose a lot of vitamins and nutrients every time you sweat. We all know that consuming too much salt is very bad for you. However the body is made up of water and salt, so just a bit of sea salt will actually cleanse your system and give you a boost in necessary vitamins. Do not just buy B vitamins when trying to create balance, buy multivitamins to get the full spectrum of what you need.

CHAPTER 8

HOW TO REDUCE YOUR APPETITE FOR SUGAR AND CARBS

"He who conquers others is strong; He who conquers himself is mighty."

- Lao Tzu

He who conquers sugar is the real master above all of this because if he can control sugar cravings, he can control almost anything. A sugar addiction is a mental addiction. Sugar cravings are a major issue not just for ketogenic eating, but any diet program. These cravings are often what throw people out of ketosis because they give into them. Sugar causes a natural production of opioids in the brain that produces a drug-like high. Many people with addiction type of personalities who choose not to abuse illegal substances may opt for sugar because of its strong pleasurable effects. Since it is a legal substance, there are no real risks of consuming it. Sugar is ok. Sugar releases that "ahh" feeling that most of us like.

Who would have ever thought that something so simple could have such a complex hold on our sanity? Well, sugar does. Its toxicity cannot be underestimated as there are many things that could go wrong in a body full of it. The obvious sign is diabetes, which could ultimately lead to other health problems and ailments such an increase in high blood pressure, which could lead to stroke, kidney disease, and foot complications. Those foot complications could lead to a limb getting amputated. More illnesses include obesity, liver disease, and cancer. The more serious effects are decaying nerves which would change the genetic makeup and molecular structure in the brain. People pumped full of sugar will normally be in a rage when prompted by external stimuli, and other behavioral issues following. The person will normally suffer from hype energy because of the sugar rush that converts into 4-5 times the fat and energy it possesses. You essentially become a superhuman, unlike Superman or Batman, but more like a marathon runner who starts off in the first place, but then finish in last because they consumed lots of energy in the beginning and ran out toward the. Think of kids getting out of school at 3 pm pumped full of sugar from vending machines and processed lunches, going out into the streets and coming back home in a hyper state and then crashing in bed to take a nap. Unfortunately, sugar eventually causes this crash, similar to the caffeine effect. Another way sugar wreaks havoc is by creating an imbalance between the essential vitamins and minerals in the body by disrupting the proper flow of calcium, magnesium, and protein into other important areas. Most obese people are addicted to sugar, which adds more bad fat in their bodies. Staying addicted to sugar could lead to other addictions such as alcoholism and drug addiction, in an attempt for the mind to feel complete. Moreover, sugar will feed cancer cells and actually cause the death of good cells, which creates more problems. Other ailments, such as food allergies and skin aging, are reasons to avoid sugar. The only remedy to prevent these things from happening is by visiting an old friend who we talked extensively about called, "a balanced diet", preferably a ketogenic diet.

It is very hard to avoid sugar because it is everywhere, disguised in many things. There is no shortage of billboards, internet ads, grocery stores, and even friends or families who are advertising food knowingly and unknowingly, full of sugar. Luckily, there are laws in this country that require food companies to list ingredients, and sugar amounts on the Nutrition Facts found on the back of most food packages. This list will help a person make better eating choices. However, advertisers have found a way around listing sugar by coming up with code names to disguise their true identity. Have you ever eaten "sugar-free" products and noticed that they still taste sweet? There are two reasons for this; they use a natural sugar alternative, which is great, or they mask the sugar with pretty names like "high fructose corn syrup", "corn starch", "dextrose", "evaporated cane juice", "fructose, agave nectar", "molasses", "barley malt", and "caramel".

Health-conscious religious people even refer to sugar as an "evil" drug with drastic effects and consequences. What makes sugar bad is not where it originates, but how it is processed. Sugar cane is a natural plant from Southeastern Asia that has a high alkaline state because of all the vitamins and minerals in it. However, sugar processing plants use refined sugar by taking sugar cane through an intricate process that strips vitamins, minerals, nutrients, and enzymes from the plant. Refined sugar normally tastes bland, just like that caramel sundae I discussed earlier, but real complex sugar has a natural sweetness that you would truly enjoy. Refined sugar is so dangerous that it literally destroys everything it touches in the body, like fire to dry tinder, and there is no stopping it when it rages and takes over. Refined sugar weakens the enamel on teeth and depletes vitamin B. The list goes on. However, it tastes "good," and that is what attracts. On the contrary, the majority of what we eat would taste plain without sugar. Ever had oatmeal without sugar? We have an association with sugar that is an intrinsic part of our being, so it is truly hard to get away from it. Now, carbs are a different story...

There are generally two types of carbs: good and bad. The "good" complex carbs are full of fiber and mostly found in whole grains such as legumes, nuts, seeds, brown rice, oats, strawberries, and bananas, just to name a few. The "bad" simple carbs, such as honey and fruit juices are notorious for disguising themselves as regular carbs, but turning into sugar once you consume them. It is advised by healthcare professionals that diabetics should not eat carb-heavy foods like white bread and French fries because they will raise the blood sugar. Let's use complex and simple carbs along the lines of white and brown rice. Brown rice (complex carbs) is natural because it is grown just the way it is, but white rice (simple carbs) is refined and stripped of most vitamins and minerals. Vegetables and fruits have the right amount of carbs we need.

I have come up with some of the top ways you can reduce your appetite for sugar and carbohydrates so that these foods are a thing of the past for you! With a little persistence, you won't even be craving toxic sugar anymore, and ketogenic living will be your new reality.

Step #1: Be Patient

Again, with the patience theme, you need to be patient with sugar cravings. Cravings only tend to last an hour or so, and no matter how intense they come on, it's important to remember that they will subside!

Give yourself an hour, distract yourself by going for a walk, or calling a friend and you may be surprised to see this craving dissipate. Sometimes cravings are very powerful urges that cannot be overcome with willpower alone. You need Herculean strength. The key to success in dieting is staying patient regardless of how you feel. Understand that those cravings will eventually pass and go away because they do not last forever. There are people who have stopped binge eating and do not crave an excessive amount of food anymore because they stayed loyal to a diet. If they can do it, so can you. There are documentaries about people who are forced to live in survival situations and almost starving to death. One common theme is how they stop feeling hungry as time passes. This is very dangerous when it happens, but shows that your body can get used to anything. Although they are forced into a survival situation where they would need to fast, and you are doing this keto diet by choice, you could learn from their success. Watch a few "I Shouldn't Be Alive" documentary shows and analyze how they switched to an immediately responsible mindset. Our bodies can withstand so many things beyond our understanding, so something as simple as keto dieting should not be hard at all. Stay patient, and the cravings will eventually go away. Some of the ways to stay more patient is to slow down a bit and take an objective look at exactly what you are doing. The voices in your head will start calling your name to eat sugar and carbs - the infamous tug-of-war between the devil and angel - and start a mental conversation like "I will eat just a little bit of junk food", "but I will only eat just one", "I need to go back to my old ways", "Forget this diet, it is horrible", "I am tired of it", "Let me go buy some pizza!" Do not give in to those thoughts and feelings. Just relax and think logically about the final goal you are trying to achieve without letting emotion dominate eating choices. Remember that dieting and weight loss is a mental game, so play to win. Go somewhere isolated and clear your mind. Collect your thoughts. And come back with both feet hitting the ground running and striving for greatness. Understand the depth of your emotions and why you are feeling them, but always stay emotionless and think logically about this diet plan. Only deviate when it is your cheat day. Patience is a necessary virtue that is very powerful once it is achieved. When you reach it, there is absolutely nothing you cannot do. Always keep the larger picture in mind. What are you working towards? What are the benefits of losing weight? What will happen if you do not diet and keep the weight on? Dig up a deeper for meaning. Understand why you want to do it. It is not about those hundreds of thousands of people paying attention to you on YouTube. It is about personal satisfaction and reaching for something on a higher level. Engage in your weight loss regimen with full speed by using the powerful virtue of patience. Learn to stay loyal, powerful, and tolerant of your diet.

Step #2: Make Healthier Alternatives

When you're just starting out, it may be hard to kick these cravings overnight, and that's ok. Create healthy alternatives such as the recipes featured in the dessert section of this book. Choose rich foods like avocado to make an avocado pudding instead of indulging in ice cream. Swap in healthier alternative and pretty soon your brain will be wired to crave the healthier version.

Step #3: Eat Frequently

One of the biggest tricks to keeping sugar cravings at bay is to eat regularly. You want to eat small but frequent meals to keep your blood sugar levels stabilized. Your body will feel more satisfied so you won't go into that starvation mode where you want to snack on all the wrong foods. It is important to eat smaller meals often and regularly, but always stay cautious about what you choose to put on your plate. In Southeastern Asian countries, there are food stalls in most places where people can walk up and have 3 meals with snacks in between per day. The island of Okinawa, Japan, have the highest life expectancies in the world because people eat frequent meals consisting of food from the nearby tropical jungles or surrounding oceans.

Step #4: Choose Whole Foods over Processed Foods

Processed foods are full of artificial junk that can cause food cravings and blood sugar imbalances. Remove the processed foods from your diet and just eat the real thing! You'll feel more satisfied, and your body will be much more nourished eating this way. It is best to always choose whole foods over processed foods for obvious reasons. We mentioned that processed foods are unnaturally pumped full of sugar and other nasty chemicals that keep you addicted and coming back for more. There is a multi-billion dollar industry advertising unnaturally processed foods daily to the billions of people living on this planet with companies selling their products off the shelves in droves. We buy processed foods all the time because we want to eat the latest brands that are constantly advertised to us. However, when you look at the sugar content and carb percentage, it is usually through the roof. But, it tastes good. Natural foods were given to us by nature for a reason, to help keep us replenished and heal us during times of illnesses. Most herbalists say that the only way to cure cancer is to simply change your diet, which will literally change your life. Physical and internal ailments would simply melt away because natural foods attack bacteria and cancers and help flush out impurities from the body that begins a healing process. Changing diet can help improve any diseases or illnesses you have, even external ones such as skin irritations. There is an entire supermarket named after whole foods, offering organic choices for people on a health kick. Look for grass-fed meats and USDA organic labels. Moreover, get familiar with healthy fats and how they work.

Step #5: Avoid Artificial Sweeteners

Even though artificial sweeteners are often seen in fad diets, they aren't recognized by the body, and your body can't differentiate between artificial sugar and regular sugar. This can lead to sugar cravings. Remove these sweeteners altogether. There are many artificial sweeteners on the market that will cause sugar and carb cravings and although there are conflicting opinions about whether artificial sweeteners would be a positive addition to a ketogenic diet, the studies show they are very dangerous to consume. Avoid aspartame and saccharin because they are full of chemical ingredients. Cravings are normal and natural, but you could consume some more protein into your diet to really fill you up. Never starve yourself and only eat when you get really hungry. Always drink enough water because the power H2O could curb your cravings for artificial sweeteners.

Step #6: Take Supplements

Some supplements can help keep sugar cravings at bay. L-glutamine, omega 3's and green tea extract are a couple of commonly used supplements. Remember always to check with your doctor before starting any new supplements. Sometimes when the body gets really hungry, it is really craving for the energy that normally comes from sugar and carbs. If you do not want to eat fruits and vegetables because you have become immune to eating processed foods and did not develop a taste for anything natural, but still want to stick to your keto diet, you could always take supplements. Some people do not trust supplements for various reasons, but if you decide to buy them it is best to choose a multivitamin to help ease the pain and get all the vitamins and minerals you need. Additionally, take fish oils to help curb those hunger feelings as well because they will actually reduce your appetite, which will aid in keeping your body in ketosis. Taking multivitamins will give you energy and give an extra boost to help absorb minerals better. A great sugar alternative substance is 500 mg L-Glutamine, which is a natural amino acid that the brain can burn for energy instead of the sugar. Supplements with B vitamins, biotin, alpha lipoic acid, zinc, vitamin E, and Chromium GTF will help regulate blood sugar. Resveratrol and Coenzyme Q10 will help get carb cravings under control and support the brain with neurotransmitter support to relieve those chewy sensations. Other great supplements include Gymnema Sylvestre, L-tryptophan, Lipase, L-Carnitine, and Acetyl-L-Carnitine. Each has different functions but the benefits are the same: to relieve sugar and carb cravings.

Step #7: Get Enough Sleep

More often than not, sleep can be the reason you crave sweet. A lack of sleep can cause your hormones to be out of whack and can lead to cravings. Be sure to get quality uninterrupted sleep every single night to promote health and prevent cravings. In some cases, ketosis will make you very sleepy or even cause insomnia. A high amount of carbs is mostly found in comfort foods and when consumed produces a relaxing feeling that makes a person want to fall asleep. However, during ketosis, some people may find themselves staying up all night. When serotonin drops you may experience sleep disturbances, so avoid this by easing into the low carb diet instead of just getting right into it. This goes back to fasting and getting your body immune to being in a ketosis state. A drastic shift in carb intake can have negative effects on your sleep patterns. So, it is best to gradually make a few small adjustments instead of just quitting cold turkey. Having sleep problems is not good when you need to take care of life's responsibilities and business issues. Moreover, also look into other possible causes of sleep problems such as sleep apnea, caffeine intake, and stress because they might be the cause of it.

Step #8: Exercise

Exercise can help ward off sugar cravings as well. Exercise raises your serotonin levels, just as a sugar binge temporarily would. And exercise will help fill a void in your body by tricking it into believing there is sugar present when there is really not. By exercising regularly, you can keep your serotonin levels up naturally and fill that void without wanting to reach for junk. Although this may sound somewhat cliché, people do not want to exercise in the Western world anymore. Even when I fast, I typically do not workout but have come to realize it is essential to losing weight, no matter what my diet is. You could just rely on dieting for a slow weight loss, but no rigorous movement would not tighten the skin back in place. Staying loyal to a low carb diet is not enough, exercise is also needed. The best way to exercise while on a ketogenic diet is to do cardiovascular workouts and heavy weight lifting.

PART 4

7-DAY KETO MEAL PLAN

CHAPTER 9

QUICK AND EASY
TO DO MEAL PLAN

*"The trouble with always trying to preserve the health of the body is that it
is so difficult to do without destroying the health of the mind."*

- G.K. Chesterton

	Day 1	Day 2	Day 3	Day 4	Day 5	Day 6	Day 7
Breakfast	Creamy peppermint shake	Berry cream cheese pancakes	Avocado and bacon boats	Decadent cocoa chia pudding	Not your average omelet	Creamy peppermint shake	Berry cream cheese pancakes
Lunch	Veggie taco wrap	Asparagus soup with Greek salad	Tomato and pepper lamb stew	Fresh chicken salad	Avocado salmon wrap	Asparagus soup with Greek salad	Fresh chicken salad
Dinner	Pesto salmon filet	Sweet BBQ pork chops with arugula tomato salad	Spicy garlic shrimp	Zesty Burger with arugula tomato salad	Garlic roasted lamb	Grilled chicken with lime sauce	Coconut chicken
Snacks	Handful of almonds	Hazelnut avocado pudding	Matcha green tea chia pudding	Raw brownie	1 ounce of hard cheese with 8 pitted olives	Nutty Fudge	2 hard-boiled eggs

**Please note that all recipes are located in the following recipe section and
that serving sizes vary depending on weight, activity level, and weight loss
goals.

PART 5

40 MOUTHWATERING KETO RECIPES

CHAPTER 10

BREAKFAST RECIPES

Decadent Cocoa Chia Pudding

This recipe is perfect for all chocolate lovers who don't want to feel guilty after a little chocolate indulgence! This chia pudding has the perfect balance of dark chocolate with a hint of coffee to get your day started on the right foot.

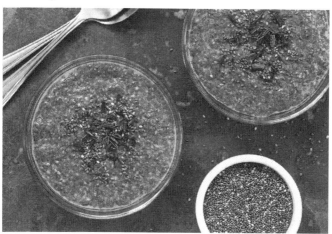

Dietary Label: (GF, V, EF, DF)
Serves: 2
Prep Time: 10 minutes & set overnight
Cook Time: 0 minutes

Ingredients:

- ¼ cup chia seeds
- ½ cup full-fat coconut milk

- 1 tsp. pure vanilla extract
- 1 drop of vanilla crème stevia extract
- 1 tsp. cocoa powder
- 1 Tbsp. Brewed and chilled coffee
- 2 Tbsp. Raw cocoa nibs (1 Tbsp. reserved for topping.)

Directions:

1. The night before you wish to enjoy this breakfast, brew a strong cup of coffee to enjoy, and reserve 1 Tbsp. for the chia pudding, and enjoy the rest of your coffee!

2. After the Tbsp. of coffee has chilled, add the coconut milk, and coffee into a mason jar, or another glass container, and stir. Add in the vanilla, stevia, and cocoa powder, and whisk. At this point, you should be drooling over cocoa and coffee aroma! This is how you know your chia pudding is going to be delicious.

3. Add in the chia seeds, and 1 Tbsp. cocoa nibs and stir to combine.

4. That's it! Now, all you need to do is refrigerate this pudding overnight and in the morning you will have magically created an amazing chia pudding breakfast full of healthy fats to get you through your morning. Top with another tablespoon of cocoa nibs in the morning, and enjoy or bring on the go!

Substitutions:

- If you have a coconut allergy, don't worry because you can easily swap in unsweetened rice milk instead! Use the same amount of rice milk to make an allergy-friendly decadent chia pudding.

- If you are not a coffee fan, you can eliminate the brewed coffee, and add an extra tablespoon of coconut milk.

Nutritional Information:

Carbohydrates: 19g
Net Carbs: 8g
Sugar: 2g
Fiber: 11g
Fats: 29g
Protein: 6g
Calories: 344

Creamy Peppermint Breakfast Shake

If you love peppermint patties, but these minty candies are a thing of the past you are going to love this smoothie. Packed with creamy and nourishing ingredients that allow you to have your milkshake and eat it too, even for breakfast!

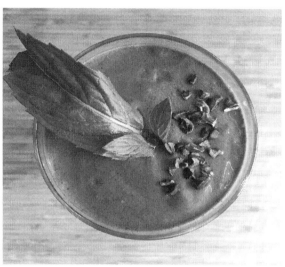

Dietary Label: (GF, V, EF, DF)
Serves: 1
Prep Time: 5 minutes
Cook Time: 0 minutes

Ingredients:

- 1 cup of unsweetened cashew milk
- 1 handful of fresh spinach
- 1 Tbsp. raw cashews
- 2 fresh mint leaves
- 1 tsp. pure vanilla extract
- 2 tsp. raw unsweetened cocoa nibs (1 tsp. reserved for topping)
- 1 scoop of unsweetened whey protein
- 1 handful of ice

Directions:

1. To make this delicious peppermint smoothie, simply add the cashew milk and cashews to the base of a blender. Next, add in the remaining ingredients, reserving 1 tsp. of the raw cocoa nibs.

2. Now, all you have to do is switch your blender on to blend! Don't be shy here, blend until super smooth.

3. Pour the creamy deliciousness into a large glass, and top with the remaining 1 tsp. of raw cocoa nibs.

4. Enjoy right away!

Substitutions:

- You can use unsweetened coconut milk in place of cashew milk if desired.
- If you love the peppermint flavor, feel free to add in an additional mint lead to enhance the peppermint flavor.

Nutritional Information:

Carbohydrates: 10g
Net Carbs: 8g
Sugar: 3g
Fiber: 2g
Fats: 14g
Protein: 27g
Calories: 261

Berry Cream Cheese Pancakes

If you've missed your weekend pancakes since going low-carb, this recipe is for you! Made without the use of any flour, these pancakes are super decadent and will hit the spot for any pancake lover.

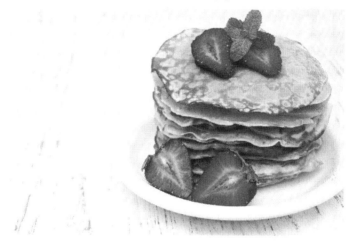

Dietary Label: (GF, EF)
Serves: 4
Prep Time: 5 minutes
Cook Time: 10 minutes

Ingredients:

- ¼ cup cream cheese
- 2 whole eggs
- 1 drop of stevia extract
- ½ tsp. ground nutmeg
- 1 tsp. pure vanilla extract
- 1 Tbsp. coconut oil for cooking
- 1 cup of fresh strawberries, halved

Directions:

1. This recipe really couldn't get any simpler, simply add all of the ingredients into a blender, or food processor and blend until smooth.

2. Next, pour the pancake mixture into a measuring cup and heat a large skillet over medium heat with the coconut oil.

3. Pour ¼ of the batter into the skillet and wait for these delicious pancakes to be ready. This typically takes about 2 minutes per side. Repeat until all of the pancakes are cooked.

4. Serve with the fresh strawberries and be amazed and how much these resemble real pancakes!

Substitutions:

- If you choose not to use eggs, you can try to use a vegan egg replacer.

- For a dairy free cream cheese substitution, choose a dairy free cream cheese, and use just as you would regular cream cheese.

Nutritional Information:

Carbohydrates: 4g
Net Carbs: 3g
Sugar: 3g
Fiber: 1g
Fats: 11g
Protein: 4g
Calories: 127

Not Your Average Veggie Omelet

If you're tired of the standard breakfast egg omelet, try this spicy loaded omelet to help spice up your breakfast a little.

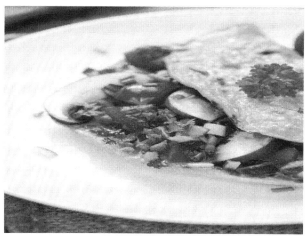

Dietary Label: (GF, DF)
Serves: 1
Prep Time: 5 minutes
Cook Time: 10 minutes

Ingredients:

- 2 whole eggs
- ¼ cup cremini mushrooms
- 1 chopped tomato
- 2 Tbsp. chopped red onion
- ½ jalapeno pepper, chopped
- 1 handful of fresh cilantro
- Salt & Pepper to taste
- 1 Tbsp. coconut oil for cooking

Directions:

1. Simply add the coconut oil into an omelet skillet over medium heat.

2. While the pan is heating, add the eggs to a mixing bowl, and whisk. Pour into the pan.

3. Cook until the eggs begin to cook, and the edges are crispy. Add in the freshly chopped veggies to one side, and fold the other side over to cover.

4. Cook for an additional 2-3 minutes each side.

5. Flip onto a plate and get ready to devour this! Season with salt and pepper if needed.

Substitutions:

- If you choose not to use eggs, you can use tofu.
- For a less spicy option, eliminate the jalapeño pepper.

Nutritional Information:

Carbohydrates: 10g
Net Carbs: 8g
Sugar: 6g
Fiber: 2g
Fats: 22g
Protein: 13g
Calories: 287

Avocado & Bacon Boat

This recipe is for anyone who loves a savory VS. sweet breakfast. Packed with delicious creamy flavors from the avocado with the perfect balance of salty goodness from the bacon. Top this with a fried egg, and you have the perfect breakfast.

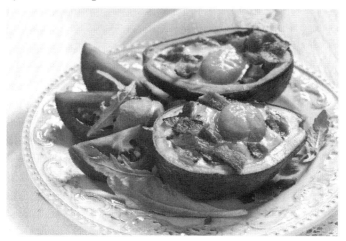

Dietary Label: (GF, DF)
Serves: 1
Prep Time: 5 minutes
Cook Time: 10 minutes

Ingredients:

- 1/2 avocado, pitted
- 2 fried eggs
- 2 slices of bacon
- ½ chopped tomato
- 1 Tbsp. coconut oil for cooking
- 1 small pinch of salt to taste

Directions:

1. After you make your fried eggs according to your liking, it's time to whip up the superstar of this recipe, the bacon. Add the bacon

to a preheated pan with the coconut oil and cook until crispy. This may take up to 20 minutes.

2. While the bacon is cooking, slice, and pit the avocado, and top each half with a fried egg. Once the bacon is done, chop into small bits, and add on top of the egg.

3. Season with a small pinch of salt if needed, and serve with a sliced tomato.

4. Enjoy this savory breakfast right away while warm!

Substitutions:

- If you choose not to use eggs, you can sub in tofu.

Nutritional Information:

Carbohydrates: 15g
Net Carbs: 10g
Sugar: 3g
Fiber: 10g
Fats: 47g
Protein: 18g
Calories: 530

CHAPTER 11

PORK RECIPES

Sautéed Rosemary Pork Chops

A delicious herb-infused pork chop recipe perfect for all pork lovers! This recipe combines the perfect combination of garlic and rosemary for a harmonious balance of pure luxury.

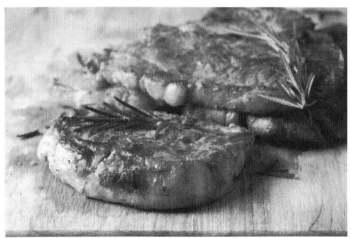

Dietary Label: (GF, EF)
Serves: 4
Prep Time: 5 minutes
Cook Time: 10 minutes

Ingredients:

- 1.5 lbs. pork chops
- 2 Tbsp. butter

- ¼ tsp. cumin
- ½ tsp. garlic powder
- 1 Tbsp. fresh rosemary springs
- 1 tsp. salt
- ½ tsp. pepper
- Tbsp. coconut oil for cooking

Directions:

1. Start by making the delicious pork rub by combining the rosemary, garlic, cumin, salt, and pepper. Rub the pork with the rub to cover completely. Don't skimp on this part!

2. In a large skillet, melt the butter and add the seasoned pork chops. Brown on both sides cooking on high, and then reduce heat to medium and cook for another 5-10 minutes each side or until cooked through.

Serving Suggestion: Enjoy with sautéed vegetables or a side of salad greens.

Substitutions:

- For a dairy-free option, use coconut oil instead of butter for cooking.

Nutritional Information:

Carbohydrates: 1g
Net Carbs: 1g
Sugar: 0g
Fiber: 0g
Fats: 17g
Protein: 29g
Calories: 278

Sweet BBQ Pork Chops

If you're a BBQ lover, these pork chops may be the perfect keto friendly recipe for you. These sweet BBQ Pork Chops are low in carbs, sugar, and bursting with traditional BBQ flavor with a subtle hint of cocoa for a unique flavor.

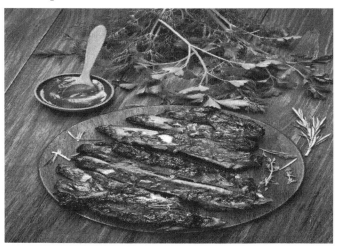

Dietary Label: (GF, EF, DF)
Serves: 4
Prep Time: 10 minutes plus marinate overnight
Cook Time: 75 minutes

Ingredients:

- 1 lb. pork ribs
- ½ white onion, diced
- 2 garlic cloves, chopped
- 1 tsp. paprika
- 2 tsp. raw unsweetened cocoa powder
- ¼ cup olive oil
- ¼ cup no added salt tomato paste
- 1 tsp. cumin
- ½ tsp. salt

- 1 pinch of black pepper
- 1 sprig of fresh rosemary for garnish

Directions:

1. To make these ribs extra tasty, it's best to prep them the night before, so mix up the marinade and let this sit in the fridge for at least 12 hours before cooking.

2. To make this zesty marinade, add all of the seasoning, raw cocoa powder, onion, garlic, olive oil, and tomato paste into a food processor, and blend. Add the pork ribs into a large baking dish, and baste with the homemade BBQ sauce. Set in the fridge overnight.

3. The next day, preheat the oven to 350 degrees F, and place the ribs into the oven, and cook for 1 hour or up to 75 minutes.

4. Garnish with fresh rosemary.

Serving Suggestions: Serve with a side of steamed vegetables, or a side salad.

Substitutions:

- If you prefer a spicier flavor, you can add a pinch of red pepper flakes, or a dash of cayenne pepper to increase the heat.
- For a savory flavor, try increasing the raw cocoa powder.

Nutritional Information:

Carbohydrates: 6g
Net Carbs: 4g
Sugar: 0g
Fiber: 2g
Fats: 27g
Protein: 14g
Calories: 324

Herb Infused Pork Tenderloin

This herb-infused pork tenderloin is perfect for family gatherings and is sure to impress. With only a handful of ingredients, you can create the most tender and flavorful low carb tenderloin in under 90 minutes!

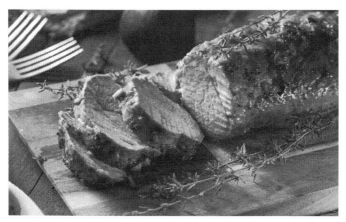

Dietary Label: (GF, EF,)
Serves: 8
Prep Time: 10 minutes plus marinate overnight
Cook Time: 75 minutes

Ingredients:

- (1) 4 lb. pork tenderloin
- 3 Tbsp. olive oil
- 2 garlic cloves, chopped
- ¼ cup chopped white onion
- 4 rosemary sprigs
- 8 thyme sprigs

Sauce

- 2 Tbsp. ghee
- 1 cup low sodium vegetable broth

- 3 tsp. Dijon mustard
- ¼ tsp. salt
- 1 pinch of black pepper

Directions:

1. To make this delicious herb-infused pork roast, start by preheating the oven to 350 degrees F.

2. Add the pork tenderloin roast into a large oven safe baking dish. Rub with the olive oil, and seasoning. Be sure to cover thoroughly! Don't skimp here; you want this roast to be bursting with flavor.

3. Roast the tenderloin for about 60 minutes, or until a thermometer inserted in the middle reads 140-145 degrees F.

4. Once the pork tenderloin is thoroughly cooked, transfer the pork onto a cutting board, and allow it to rest for about 20 minutes. Keep in mind that the temperature will increase as the pork rests.

5. While the pork is resting, mix up the creamy sauce. Add all of the sauce ingredients together in a small stock pot, and stir until melted.

6. Remove the whole herbs from the pork, and pour the sauce over the cooked pork tenderloin.

7. Slice and enjoy!

Serving Suggestions: Serve with oven roasted garlic asparagus or steamed broccoli.

Substitutions:

- Feel free to add in any of your other favor herbs of choice to alter the flavor according to your taste.
- For a dairy-free option, use vegan butter instead of ghee.

Nutritional Notes:

- Depending on the marinating time, cook time, etc. the amount of marinade consumed will vary. The nutritional information reflects the full amount of each marinade ingredient.

Nutritional Information:

Carbohydrates: 1g
Net Carbs: 1g
Sugar: 0g
Fiber: 0g
Fats: 22g
Protein: 25g
Calories: 304

CHAPTER 12

CHICKEN RECIPES

Grilled Chicken with Lime Sauce

If you're tired of the traditionally grilled chicken breast, this grilled lime chicken breast will blow you away! With just a couple of ingredients, you can spice up the traditional chicken breast to something new and exciting.

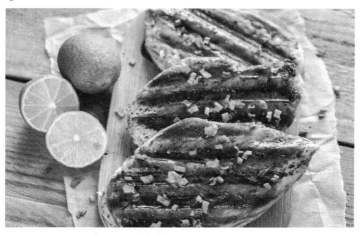

Dietary Label: (GF, EF, DF)
Serves: 4
Prep Time: 10 minutes + 60 minutes marinating time
Cook Time: 15 minutes

Ingredients:

- 4 boneless, skinless chicken breasts
- 1 finely chopped scallion

- 1 garlic clove, chopped
- 3 Tbsp. reduced-sodium soy sauce
- 1 Tbsp. olive oil
- 2 tsp. freshly squeezed lime juice
- ½ Tbsp. honey

Directions:

1. In a large and shallow baking dish, add the lime sauce ingredients: Reduced-sodium soy sauce, olive oil, chopped garlic, freshly squeezed lime juice, and honey. Mix to combine, and add the chicken breast, toss to cover. Place in the refrigerator and marinate for 30-60 minutes.

2. Right before the chicken is finished marinating, preheat a grill outside.

3. Once the chicken has marinated, grill for about 8 minutes each side or until the juices run clear and both sides are browned.

4. Garnish with freshly chopped scallions.

5. That's it! Enjoy right away.

Serving Suggestions: Enjoy with a salad, or alone with some grilled vegetables.

Substitutions:

- Feel free to add in any of your other favor herbs of choice to alter the flavor according to your taste.
- For a dairy-free option, use vegan butter instead of ghee.

Nutritional Notes:

- Depending on the marinating time, cook time, etc. the amount of marinade consumed will vary. The nutritional information reflects the full amount of each marinade ingredient.

Nutritional Information:

Carbohydrates: 3g
Net Carbs: 3g
Sugar: 2g

Fiber: 0g
Fats: 7g
Protein: 27g
Calories: 185

Maple & Mustard Grilled Chicken

A sweet and salty chicken recipe that won't cause you a ton of carbs or sugar! This is a perfect option for summer grilling, and pairs wonderfully with a salad to add a nice protein punch and added flavor.

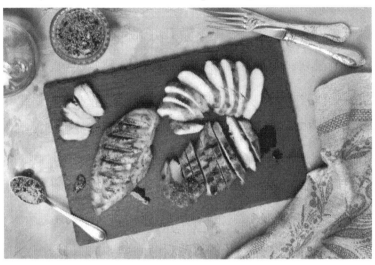

Dietary Label: (GF, EF, DF)
Serves: 4
Prep Time: 10 minutes + 30 minutes marinating time
Cook Time: 15 minutes

Ingredients:

- 4 boneless, skinless chicken breasts
- ¼ cup olive oil
- 3 Tbsp. spicy Dijon mustard
- 3 Tbsp. reduced-sodium soy sauce
- 1 Tbsp. pure maple syrup
- 1 tsp. garlic powder
- 1 tsp. apple cider vinegar
- Fresh cilantro for garnish

Directions:

1. To make the maple marinade, simply add the olive oil, mustard, soy sauce, maple, garlic powder, and apple cider vinegar into a medium sized mixing bowl, and whisk.

2. Next, add the chicken breasts to a glass baking dish, and cover with the maple marinade. Allow this to sit in the fridge for 30 minutes for best results.

3. Preheat the grill, and grill each marinated chicken breast for about 8 minutes each side or until the juices run clear.

4. Garnish with fresh cilantro, and enjoy!

Serving Suggestions: This chicken pairs wonderfully with a salad, and some balsamic dressing.

Substitutions:

- To make this a little extra spicy, add in some red pepper flakes.
- For a vegetarian option, you can use the same marinade for tempeh.

Nutritional Notes:

- Depending on the marinating time, cook time, etc. the amount of marinade consumed will vary. The nutritional information reflects the full amount of each marinade ingredient.

Nutritional Information:

Carbohydrates: 5g
Net Carbs: 5g
Sugar: 4g
Fiber: 0g
Fats: 17g
Protein: 27g
Calories: 284

Coconut Chicken

If you love the flavor and texture of breaded chicken, you're going to love this tropical infused chicken breast crisp with shredded coconut for the perfect balance of sweet and savory.

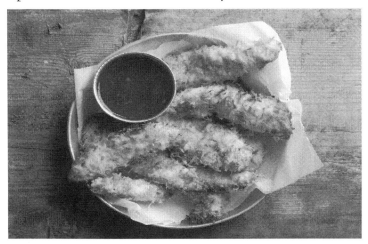

Dietary Label: (GF, DF)
Serves: 4
Prep Time: 30 minutes
Cook Time: 15 minutes

Ingredients:

- 4 boneless, skinless chicken breasts cut into strips
- 2 cups of unsweetened shredded coconut
- 1/4 cup cornstarch
- 3 eggs, beaten
- Pinch of salt & pepper
- 3 Tbsp. Coconut oil for frying

Directions:

1. Start by preheating a large skillet with coconut oil over medium heat.

2. While the pan is heating up, mix the cornstarch, salt, and pepper in a mixing bowl, and set aside. Crack the eggs into a separate mixing bowl and whisk. In a third bowl, add the shredded coconut.

3. Take the chicken, and dip it into the cornstarch mix followed by the egg mix and finally the shredded coconut.

4. Add to the heated pan, and fry on both sides for about 4-5 minutes or until crispy and cooked through. You will know the chicken is done when the center is no longer pink, and you want the coconut shreds to be crispy and golden brown.

5. Enjoy with a side of hot chili sauce.

Serving Suggestions: Enjoy this coconut chicken tossed in salads or served as an appetizer with a spritz of freshly squeezed lemon or orange juice for a tangy flavor.

Substitutions:

- Use almond flour in place of the coconut shreds for a more traditional breaded chicken.
- Use a vegan egg replacer for the eggs for an egg-free option.

Nutritional Notes:

- Depending on the cook time, the size of the chicken, etc. the amount of coconut oil consumed will vary. The nutritional information reflects the full amount of the coconut oil listed.

Nutritional Information:

Carbohydrates: 14g
Net Carbs: 10g
Sugar: 3g
Fiber: 4g
Fats: 30g
Protein: 31g
Calories: 445

Almond Crusted Chicken

A perfect alternative to traditionally breaded chicken. A delicious low carb option full of rich and savory flavors serving with a spicy dip.

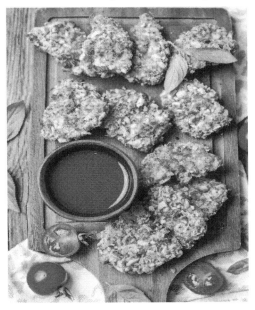

Dietary Label: (GF, DF)
Serves: 6
Prep Time: 30 minutes
Cook Time: 15 minutes

Ingredients:

- 4 boneless, skinless chicken breasts cut in half
- 2 cups of blanched almonds, ground into a fine almond flour
- 3 eggs, beaten
- ¼ tsp. paprika
- Pinch of salt & pepper
- 3 Tbsp. Coconut oil for frying
- ½ cup canned tomatoes, blended
- 2 Tbsp. hot sauce

Directions:

1. Start by preheating a large skillet with coconut oil over medium heat.

2. While the pan is heating up, crack the eggs into a separate mixing bowl and whisk. Add the salt, pepper, and cayenne pepper. In a third bowl, add the homemade almond flour

3. Take the chicken, and dip it into the egg mix and finally the ground almonds.

4. Add to the heated pan, and fry on both sides for about 4-5 minutes or until crispy and cooked through. You will know the chicken is done when the center is no longer pink.

5. While the chicken is cooking, add the canned tomatoes, and hot sauce to a food processor or blender and blend until super smooth.

6. Serve the cooked chicken with the hot tomato sauce.

Serving Suggestions: Enjoy this almond chicken as an appetizer or alongside steamed vegetables.

Substitutions:

- Reduce the amount of hot sauce for a less spicy option.
- Use a vegan egg replacer for the eggs for an egg-free option.

Nutritional Notes:

- Depending on the cook time, the size of the chicken, etc. the amount of coconut oil consumed will vary. The nutritional information reflects the full amount of the coconut oil listed.

Nutritional Information:

Carbohydrates: 11g
Net Carbs: 4g
Sugar: 3g
Fiber: 7g
Fats: 35g
Protein: 31g
Calories: 466

CHAPTER 13

FISH & SEAFOOD RECIPES

Spicy Garlic Shrimp

If you love shrimp scampi, this spicy garlic shrimp recipe takes things to a whole new level! With basil, olive oil, and crushed garlic this recipe slightly resembles a shrimp scampi with a new healthy spin.

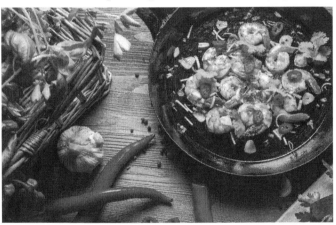

Dietary Label: (SF, GF, DF, EF)
Serves: 3
Prep Time: 15 minutes
Cook Time: 10 minutes

Ingredients:

- 18 deveined large shrimp
- 3 garlic cloves, chopped
- 1 scallion, chopped

- ½ jalapeno pepper, chopped
- 3 Tbsp. olive oil
- 1 Tbsp. ghee
- 1 handful fresh cilantro
- ¼ tsp. sea salt

Directions:

1. To make this new and improved keto shrimp scampi recipe, add the olive oil to a large skillet with the shrimp. Cook until the shrimp turns pink and the tails begin to curl.

2. Add the chopped garlic, scallion, pepper, and ghee. Sauté for another 3-5 minute. Turn off the heat and toss in the cilantro, and ¼ tsp. salt.

3. Enjoy right away!

Serving Suggestions: Enjoy this spicy garlic shrimp with a Spiralized zucchini for a low carb pasta dish.

Substitutions:

- Remove the jalapeno pepper and swap in a bell pepper for a less spicy option.

Nutritional Information:

Carbohydrates: 2g
Net Carbs: 2g
Sugar: 0g
Fiber: 0g
Fats: 18g
Protein: 6g
Calories: 196

Pesto Salmon Filet

A delicious basil infused salmon filet with traditional Italian flavors without the extra carbs! Full of healthy fats to keep you full and full of energy all day, this is the perfect pick me up for lunch or dinner recipe.

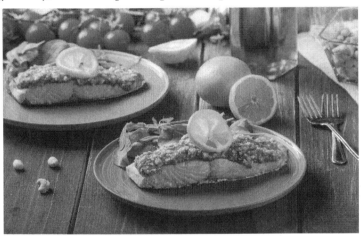

Dietary Label: (SF, GF, DF, EF)
Serves: 4
Prep Time: 20 minutes
Cook Time: 10 minutes

Ingredients:

- 4 (3 ounces) wild caught salmon filets
- 2 Tbsp. freshly squeezed lemon juice
- 2 Tbsp. olive oil
- 1 pinch of salt & pepper
- 2 cups of fresh arugula for serving

Pesto

- ½ cup olive oil
- 2 Tbsp. freshly squeezed lemon juice
- ¼ cup pine nuts

- 1 cup packed basil
- 2 garlic cloves, peeled
- ¼ tsp. sea salt

Directions:

1. To make this delicious Italian-flavored dish start by preheating the oven to 400 degrees F.

2. Rinse the salmon fillet, remove skin if necessary and pat dry. Season with salt and pepper and add to an oven safe baking dish. Drizzle with the olive oil and lemon juice. Bake for 15-30 minutes or until the fish flakes easily with a fork.

3. While the salmon is cooking, make the pesto by adding all of the pesto ingredients to a blender or food processor and blend until smooth. Disrepute evenly among the 4 salmon filets.

Serving Suggestions: Serve with fresh arugula. You can sauté the arugula if desired.

Substitutions:

- Remove the lemon juice from the salmon marinates for a less citrusy flavor.

Nutritional Information:

Carbohydrates: 3g
Net Carbs: 2g
Sugar: 1g
Fiber: 1g
Fats: 43g
Protein: 16g
Calories: 457

Garlic Lemon Scallop

A low carb delicious lemon garlic scallop recipe that pairs wonderfully with sautéed spinach, or steamed broccoli or enjoyed alone. The lemon garlic sauce is a perfect creamy addition to this recipe.

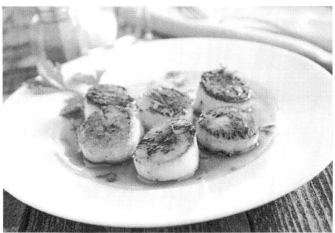

Dietary Label: (SF, GF, EF)
Serves: 6
Prep Time: 20 minutes
Cook Time: 10 minutes

Ingredients:

- 2 pounds of scallops
- ½ cup of butter
- 2 Tbsp. freshly squeezed lemon juice
- 3 garlic cloves, chopped
- ½ tsp. salt
- ¼ tsp. black pepper

Directions:

1. To make this creamy recipe, melt the butter in a large skillet over medium heat and add the garlic. Sauté for 2-3 minutes until there is a delicious garlic aroma. Add the scallops and cook for about 5-

6 minutes each side and then flip. Cook until the scallops are opaque and firm.

2. Place the scallops onto a serving plate, and add the lemon juice, salt, and pepper to the butter mixture. Whisk to combine.

3. Pour the butter garlic sauce over the scallops and split into 6 servings.

Serving Suggestions: Serve alone or with sautéed spinach.

Substitutions:

- Swap out the dairy butter for vegan butter for a dairy free option.

Nutritional Information:

Carbohydrates: 5g
Net Carbs: 5g
Sugar: 0g
Fiber: 0g
Fats: 16g
Protein: 16g
Calories:222

Coconut Shrimp

A low carb recipe that will take you to the tropics! This low-carb coconut shrimp recipe is bursting with coconut flavor and is an excellent appetizer dipped in the chili dipping sauce or served alongside a meal.

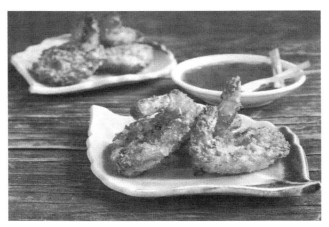

Dietary Label: (SF, GF, DF)
Serves: 6
Prep Time: 20 minutes
Cook Time: 15 minutes

Ingredients:

- 1lb of shrimp peeled and deveined
- 2 eggs, gently whisked
- 1 cup of unsweetened shredded coconut
- 1 Tbsp. coconut flour
- ¼ tsp. salt

Dip:

- ½ cup olive oil
- 2 Tbsp. red wine vinegar
- 1 Tbsp. lime juice
- 1 small red chili diced

Directions:

1. To make this tropical tasting coconut shrimp recipe, preheat the oven to 375 degrees F, and line a baking sheet with parchment paper.

2. While the oven is heating up, add the eggs into a mixing bowl and gently whisk, add the salt. In a separate bowl, add in the unsweetened shredded coconut and the coconut flour in a separate bowl.

3. Dip the shrimp into the coconut flour, then the egg mixture, and finally, the shredded coconut being sure to cover both sides.

4. Evenly distribute onto the baking sheet, and bake for about 15 minutes. Flip over and cook for another 5 minutes.

5. While those tasty shrimp are cooking, whisk up the dip by adding all of the ingredients into a mixing bowl, and whisk.

6. Enjoy the shrimp with the chili dip.

Serving Suggestions: Serve alone with the dip or to accompany a meal.

Substitutions:

- Swap out the egg for a vegan egg for a vegan option.

Nutritional Information:

Carbohydrates: 4g
Net Carbs: 2g
Sugar: 1g
Fiber: 2g
Fats: 25g
Protein: 13g
Calories: 288

CHAPTER 14

VEGETARIAN RECIPES

Greek Salad

A light and refreshing salad bursting with traditional Greek flavors. This low-carb salad option is perfect for a hot summer day or a light lunch.

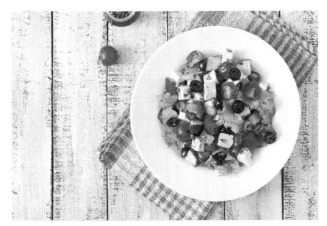

Dietary Label: (GF, DF, EF, V)
Serves: 1
Prep Time: 10 minutes
Cook Time: 5 minutes

Ingredients:

- 1 cup of romaine lettuce
- 8 grape tomatoes, sliced in half
- 4 black olive pitted and sliced

- 4 ounces of tofu, cubed
- 1 Tbsp. of fresh rosemary
- 2 Tbsp. chopped red onion
- 1 Tbsp. olive oil
- 1 Tbsp. coconut oil for cooking

Directions:

1. Start by sautéing the cubed tofu in a medium skillet with coconut oil. Cook for about 5 minutes each side or until browned. You can cook the tofu as you desire. If you prefer it crispy, cook for a few more minutes.

2. Add the lettuce into a large bowl, and top with the tomatoes, olives, red onion, rosemary, and cooked tofu. Drizzle with the olive oil.

3. Enjoy right away!

Serving Suggestions: Serve with a spritz of lemon juice for a citrus flare.

Substitutions:

- Use cilantro or parsley in place of the rosemary if desired.

Nutritional Information:

Carbohydrates: 9g
Net Carbs: 5g
Sugar: 3g
Fiber: 4g
Fats: 36g
Protein: 13g
Calories: 389

Portobello Burger

If you love a good burger and are looking for a hearty and delicious vegetarian option, this is the burger for you! The Portobello mushrooms amazingly resemble hamburger meat. Top it off with traditional burger toppings, and you have yourself a winner.

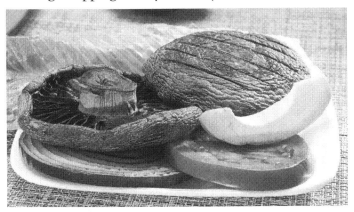

Dietary Label: (GF, DF, EF, V)
Serves: 2
Prep Time: 10 minutes
Cook Time: 10 minutes

Ingredients:

- 2 large Portobello mushroom caps
- 3 Tbsp. balsamic vinegar
- ¼ tsp. salt
- ¼ tsp. black pepper
- 1 Tbsp. coconut oil for cooking

Toppings:

- ½ red onion, sliced
- 1 avocado, pitted and sliced
- 1 plum tomato, sliced
- 2 romaine lettuce leaves

Directions:

1. Start by preheating a grill or a large slotted skillet.

2. Whisk the balsamic vinegar together with the salt and pepper, slice the mushroom stems off, and dip the mushroom caps into the marinade for 2-3 minutes.

3. Grill or sauté with coconut oil for about 5-7 minutes each side.

4. Serve with all the burger goods!

5. Enjoy as you would a traditional burger, but use the lettuce leaf for the bun.

Serving Suggestions: Serve with a side salad, or with steamed vegetables.

Substitutions:

- Add in some heat for a spicier burger if desired. Try adding paprika or cayenne to the balsamic vinegar.
- Nutritional Notes:
- Depending on the cook time, the size of the mushrooms, etc. the amount of coconut oil consumed will vary if choose to sauté the mushrooms. The nutritional information reflects the full amount of the coconut oil listed.

Nutritional Information:

Carbohydrates: 17g
Net Carbs: 10g
Sugar: 8g
Fiber: 7g
Fats: 17g
Protein: 4g
Calories: 225

Tofu Southwest Bowl

A delicious traditional southwest bowl vegetarian style! Full of nourishing veggies and a kick of cilantro for a bowl that is bursting with taco flavoring without the carbs.

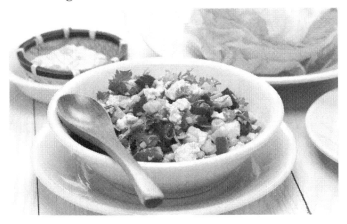

Dietary Label: (GF, DF, EF, V)
Serves: 3
Prep Time: 10 minutes
Cook Time: 10 minutes

Ingredients:

- 2 cups of romaine lettuce, chopped
- ¼ cup of canned corn rinsed and drained
- 1 tomato, chopped
- 1 red bell pepper, chopped
- 4 ounces of crumbled tofu
- 1 Tbsp. olive oil
- ¼ cup fresh cilantro
- 1 tsp. red pepper flakes
- ½ tsp. coriander
- ½ tsp. salt
- ¼ tsp. black pepper
- 1 Tbsp. coconut oil for cooking

Directions:

1. To get started, add the coconut oil into a medium sized skillet and sauté the crumbled tofu for 7-10 minutes.

2. While the tofu is cooking, add the chopped romaine lettuce to the bottom of a large bowl, and top with all the yummy veggies. Add in the seasoning, cilantro, and olive oil. Toss to combine, and top with the cooked tofu.

3. Enjoy warm or chilled.

Serving Suggestions: Serve with lettuce cups for a more traditional "taco" if desired.

Substitutions:

- Swap out the tofu and add in extra vegetables for a soy-free option.

Nutritional Information:

Carbohydrates: 10g
Net Carbs: 6g
Sugar: 4g
Fiber: 4g
Fats: 12g
Protein: 6g
Calories: 156

CHAPTER 15

BEEF & LAMB RECIPES

Zesty Burger

A traditional burger with a zesty twist, low carb style! This burger brings flavor and nutrition without the excess carbs. Now you can satisfy your burger cravings without the guilt.

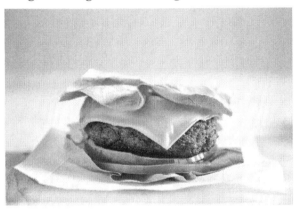

Dietary Label: (GF, DF, EF)
Serves: 4
Prep Time: 10 minutes
Cook Time: 10 minutes

Ingredients:

- 1lb of grass-fed ground beef
- 2 tsp. red pepper flakes
- ¼ tsp. cayenne pepper
- 1 Tbsp. Italian seasoning

- 1 Tbsp. reduced-sodium soy sauce
- ½ cup chopped cilantro

Serving:

- 8 butterhead lettuce leaves
- 1 sliced tomato
- 1 sliced onion
- 4 sliced of American cheese

Directions:

1. Start by preheating the oven to 350 degrees F, and lining a baking sheet with parchment paper.

2. To make this low-carb burger, add all of the burger ingredients into a large mixing bowl, and mix to combine. Form 4 large burger patties, and place on the parchment-lined baking sheet. Bake for 20 minutes, flipping halfway through or until the burger has reached the desired doneness.

3. Serve each burger with 2 lettuce leaves as the "bun" and top with the tomato, onion, and 1 slice of American cheese.

Serving Suggestions: Serve with mustard if desired.

Substitutions:

- Swap out the red pepper flakes and cayenne for a less spicy burger.

Nutritional Information:

Carbohydrates: 7g
Net Carbs: 5g
Sugar: 0g
Fiber: 2g
Fats: 21g
Protein: 26g
Calories: 322

Tomato & Pepper Lamb Stew

A quick and easy lamb stew for a savory dinner packed full of spice. If you love spicy food this recipe is for you, and is packed full of wholesome foods.

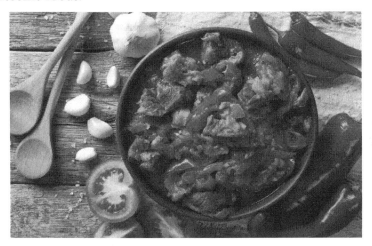

Dietary Label: (GF, DF, EF)
Serves: 5
Prep Time: 10 minutes
Cook Time: 2 hours

Ingredients:

- 3 lbs. boneless lamb cut into 2-inch chunks
- 2 cups beef stock
- 1 red pepper, cut into strips
- 1 red hot pepper, chopped
- 2 tomatoes, chopped
- 3 cloves of garlic, minced
- 1 white onion, chopped
- 1 tsp. salt
- ½ tsp. black pepper
- 1 Tbsp. coconut oil

Directions:

1. To start, add the lamb into a medium skillet with the coconut oil and sauté until brown. Add a slow-cooker with the remaining ingredients.

2. Cook on high for 2 hours. That's it, now all you need to do is wait, and smell the amazing aroma coming from the slow cooker!

3. Split into 5 servings, and enjoy!

Serving Suggestions: Serve with a side of steamed cauliflower or cauliflower rice.

Substitutions:

- Swap out the red hot pepper for a less spicy version.

Nutritional Information:

Carbohydrates: 7g
Net Carbs: 5g
Sugar: 4g
Fiber: 2g
Fats: 24g
Protein: 24g
Calories: 343

Garlic Roasted Lamb

The perfect balance of citrus yet savory this garlic roasted lamb is easy to make and has a hint of lemon with a lot of garlic! If you're a garlic lover, try this roasted lamb recipe.

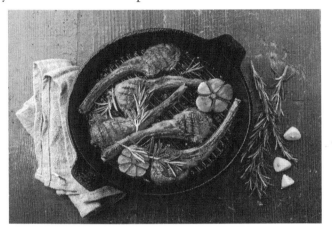

Dietary Label: (GF, DF, EF)
Serves: 4
Prep Time: 10 minutes plus chilling time overnight
Cook Time: 10 minutes

Ingredients:

- 8 lamb chops
- 4 cloves of garlic
- 1 Tbsp. freshly squeezed lemon juice
- 2 Tbsp. olive oil
- 2 tsp. freshly chopped rosemary
- 1 ½ tsp. salt
- 1 tsp. black pepper

Directions:

1. To start, you will want to make the marinade for the lamb chops. Add the garlic, lemon juice, olive oil, rosemary, salt, and pepper into a food processor. Process until smooth, and set aside.

2. Add the lamb chops onto a parchment lined baking sheet, and cover with the marinade, cover and refrigerate overnight.

3. The next day, remove the garlic marinated lamb chops from the fridge and preheat a broiler. Broil lamb for about 5 minutes each side or until they reach the desired doneness.

4. Serve 3 chops per serving, and enjoy!

Serving Suggestions: Serve with a side of steamed cauliflower or cauliflower rice.

Substitutions:

- Add in any seasoning of choice to adjust the recipe to your liking.

Nutritional Information:

Carbohydrates: 1g
Net Carbs: 1g
Sugar: 0g
Fiber: 0g
Fats: 39g
Protein: 36g
Calories: 511

CHAPTER 16

WRAPS

Turkey Lettuce Wrap

If your keto diet has you missing carbs, don't worry because this turkey lettuce wrap closely resembles the gluten loaded wraps you used to enjoy while packing in health benefits instead!

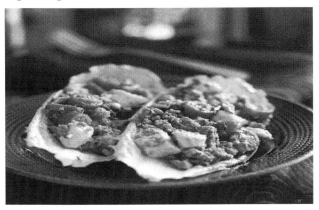

Dietary Label: (GF, DF, EF)
Serves: 4
Prep Time: 15 minutes
Cook Time: 10 minutes

Ingredients:

- 1 lb. of organic ground turkey
- 1 tsp. ground cumin
- 1 tsp. garlic powder
- 1 cup of cherry tomatoes, sliced in half

- 1 cup cubed avocado
- ½ cup of fresh cilantro
- 8 large lettuce leaves for serving
- 1 Tbsp. coconut oil for cooking

Directions:

1. Start by preheating a large skillet over medium heat with the coconut oil. Add in the ground turkey and sauté for about 5-10 minutes or until thoroughly cooked through. Add the cumin, and garlic powder.

2. Next, add in the remaining ingredients, minus the lettuce leaves and gently stir.

3. Add 2 lettuce leaves per plate, and scoop the turkey mixture onto the lettuce leaf to form a lettuce wrap.

4. Enjoy two wraps per serving!

Serving Suggestions: Serve with a dollop of sour cream or unsweetened plain Greek yogurt for topping.

Substitutions:

- Swap out the cilantro for parsley if desired, and use grass-fed ground beef in place of the turkey if desired.

Nutritional Information:

Carbohydrates: 7g
Net Carbs: 3g
Sugar: 1g
Fiber: 4g
Fats: 11g
Protein: 27g
Calories:226

Asian Fusion Pork Wrap

If you love a good Asian fusion styled wrap, you will love this new low-carb twist. With ginger flavors and freshly chopped veggies, this recipe is bursting with flavor and keeps your carbs low so you can enjoy these wraps without feeling guilty about it.

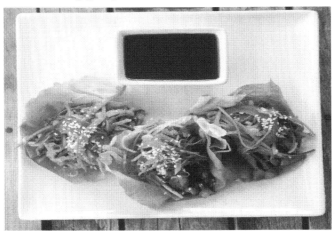

Dietary Label: (GF, DF, EF)
Serves: 2
Prep Time: 20 minutes
Cook Time: 10 minutes

Ingredients:

- 4 large butterhead lettuce leaves
- ½ purple onion, thinly sliced
- 2 scallions, chopped
- ¼ cup thinly sliced carrots
- 1 Tbsp. sesame seeds
- ½ lb. of pork, cut into strips
- 1 Tbsp. coconut oil for cooking

Sauce:

- ¼ cup reduced-sodium soy sauce

- 1 tsp. sesame oil
- 1 tsp. freshly ground ginger

Directions:

1. To start, add the coconut oil into a medium skillet with the sliced pork chops and cook for about 6-8 minutes each side or until cooked through.

2. Add the sliced red onions into the skillet, and sauté until translucent.

3. Add the lettuce leaves onto two separate plates, and fill with the cooked pork, red onions, scallions, and top with the sliced carrots and sesame seed.

4. To make the dipping sauce, simply add all of the sauce ingredients together in a mixing bowl, and whisk. Serve with the Asian fusion lettuce wraps, and enjoy!

Serving Suggestions: Serve with a side of steamed veggies for an added health kick.

Substitutions:

- Swap out the reduced-sodium soy sauce for coconut aminos for a soy-free option.

Nutritional Information:

Carbohydrates: 10g
Net Carbs: 7g
Sugar: 0g
Fiber: 3g
Fats: 21g
Protein: 18g
Calories: 289

Vegetarian Taco Wrap

If you're looking for a way to enjoy tacos without the meat, here is a vegetarian taco wrap that will hit the spot! With a hint of zesty flare, this wrap recipe has the authentic flavors that come with the traditional taco, but formed into a wrap instead.

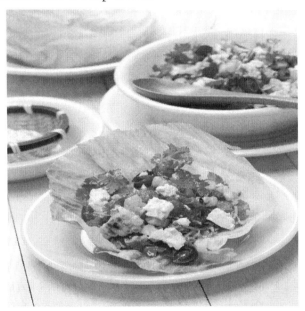

Dietary Label: (GF, DF, EF, V)
Serves: 2
Prep Time: 15 minutes
Cook Time: 10 minutes

Ingredients:

- 4 large butterhead lettuce leaves
- 1 cup of crumbled tofu
- ¼ cup of corn
- 1 hot red pepper, sliced
- 1 handful of fresh cilantro
- 1 Tbsp. coconut oil

Directions:

1. To make this deliciously simple recipe, simply add the coconut oil into a large skillet with the crumbled tofu and cook for about 7 minutes. Add in the corn, and cook for another 2-3 minutes or until the corn is lightly browned.

2. Evenly split the tofu and corn mixture among 4 large lettuce leaves, and top with the hot red pepper, and fresh cilantro.

3. Enjoy!

Serving Suggestions: Serve with a dollop of sour cream.

Substitutions:

- Swap out the red hot pepper for a less spicy version.

Nutritional Information:

Carbohydrates: 8g
Net Carbs: 6g
Sugar: 2g
Fiber: 2g
Fats: 15g
Protein: 14g
Calories: 198

Avocado Salmon Wrap

A unique variation to the standard wrap recipe. This avocado salmon wrap comes packed with healthy fats and omega-3's for a healthy balanced lunch or afternoon snack. This recipe is perfect for salmon lovers!

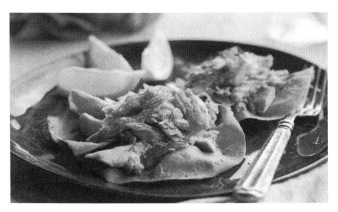

Dietary Label: (GF, DF, EF, SF)
Serves: 2
Prep Time: 15 minutes
Cook Time: 10 minutes

Ingredients:

- 4 large butterhead lettuce leaves
- 3-ounce wild-caught salmon filet
- 1 Tbsp. freshly squeezed lemon juice
- ½ cup cubed avocado
- 2 tsp. fresh dill
- ½ tsp. sea salt
- 1 Tbsp. coconut oil for cooking

Directions:

1. To start, add the coconut oil into a medium skillet with the salmon, and sauté for 7-10 minutes or until cooked through. Season with the sea salt, lemon juice, and dill.

2. Evenly split the salmon mixture among 4 lettuce wraps, and top with freshly sliced avocado.

3. Split into 2 servings and enjoy right away!

Serving Suggestions: Serve with a side of steamed broccoli, or enjoy as a mid-day snack for an added dose of omega-3's and protein.

Substitutions:

- Use tuna in place of the salmon if desired.

Nutritional Information:

Carbohydrates: 5g
Net Carbs: 2g
Sugar: 1g
Fiber: 3g
Fats: 15g
Protein: 10g
Calories: 186

CHAPTER 17

SIDE DISHES

Roasted Veggies for Two

A quick and easy side dish for two. These roasted vegetables pair perfectly with just about any dish and make for a perfect healthy addition to pair with a hearty protein.

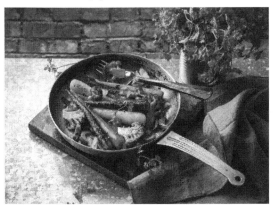

Dietary Label: (GF, DF, EF, V)
Serves: 2
Prep Time: 5 minutes
Cook Time: 5 minutes

Ingredients:

- 4 large rainbow colored carrots
- ½ red onion, thinly sliced
- 1 cup of broccoli florets
- 1 tsp. sea salt

- ½ tsp. black pepper
- 2 Tbsp. coconut oil

Directions:

1. To make this easy and delicious dish, add the coconut oil into a large skillet over medium heat.

2. Wash the carrots, and broccoli and slice the onions and add to the skillet. Sauté for 3-5 minutes until the veggies are brown and the onions are translucent.

Serving Suggestions: Serve alongside any meal. These veggies pair great with baked or roasted chicken or alongside a salmon filet.

Substitutions:

- Add in extra spices and adjust according to your taste.

Nutritional Information:

Carbohydrates: 17g
Net Carbs: 12g
Sugar: 8g
Fiber: 5g
Fats: 14g
Protein: 3g
Calories: 193

Lemon-Roasted Green Beans

A lemony garlic infused green bean dish that pairs perfectly with a flank steak or a grilled chicken dish. Low in carbs but bursting flavor.

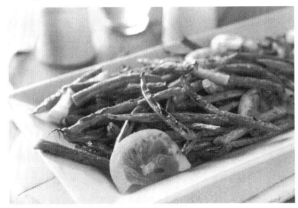

Dietary Label: (GF, EF)
Serves: 2
Prep Time: 5 minutes
Cook Time: 10 minutes

Ingredients:

- 1 bunch of green beans
- 2 Tbsp. freshly squeezed lemon juice
- 2 garlic cloves, chopped
- 1 lemon, quartered
- 1 Tbsp. butter

Directions:

1. Simply bring a large pot of water to a boil, and add in the quartered lemon, and the green beans. Boil for 5 minutes, drain and rinse.

2. Add the butter to a skillet over low heat and add in the cooked green beans, and garlic. Sauté for about 3 minutes.

3. Add the green beans into a serving bowl, and drizzle with the freshly squeezed lemon juice.

Serving Suggestions: Serve with a hamburger or veggie burger.

Substitutions:

- Swap out the butter for coconut oil for a dairy-free option.

Nutritional Information:

Carbohydrates: 7g
Net Carbs: 5g
Sugar: 0g
Fiber: 2g
Fats: 6g
Protein: 1g
Calories: 78

Cabbage Slaw

A low carb slaw that pair perfectly with a low carb wrap or to serve as an appetizer at your next dinner party. This recipe is truly guilt free, and super light for the hotter summer months.

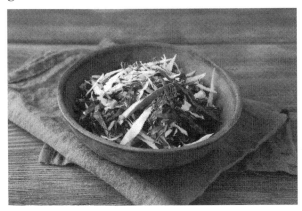

Dietary Label: (GF, EF, DF, V)
Serves: 5
Prep Time: 10 minutes
Cook Time: 0 minutes

Ingredients:

- 1 medium red cabbage thinly sliced
- ½ cup of fresh dill
- ½ of a red onion, thinly sliced
- 2 Tbsp. red wine vinegar
- 1 Tbsp. olive oil
- 1 tsp. sea salt
- 1 tsp. black pepper

Directions:

1. To make this super simple slaw, add all of the ingredients into a mixing bowl, and toss to combine.

2. That's it! You now have yourself a delicious guilt-free appetizer everyone can love!

Serving Suggestions: Serve with a keto style wrap or alongside of a keto style burger or veggie burger.

Substitutions:

- Add in garlic for an added kick.

Nutritional Information:

Carbohydrates: 7g
Net Carbs: 4g
Sugar: 4g
Fiber: 2g
Fats: 3g
Protein: 1g
Calories: 56

Creamed Spinach

If you love creamed spinach, you will love this recipe. This is the perfect dip for veggies, or to serve with a keto style wrap.

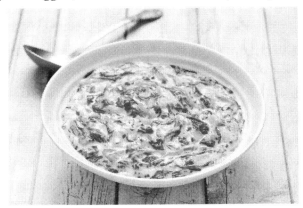

Dietary Label: (GF, EF)
Serves: 10
Prep Time: 5 minutes
Cook Time: 0 minutes

Ingredients:

- 1 cup of fresh spinach
- 1 shallot, chopped
- ½ cup whipped cream cheese
- ½ cup of cottage cheese
- 1 Tbsp. freshly squeeze lime juice
- 2 cloves of garlic, chopped
- 1 tsp. salt
- ½ tsp. black pepper

Directions:

1. This recipe is super easy to make, and only takes about 5 minutes of your time! All you need to do is place all of the ingredients into the base of a food processor, and blend until smooth.

2. Serve right away, or chill for a few hours before serving.

3. Enjoy at your next dinner party for a delicious appetizer!

Serving Suggestions: Serve with chopped veggies or serve as a dip for a keto style wrap.

Substitutions:

- Add in chopped onion for an added kick of flavor.

Nutritional Information:

Carbohydrates: 1g
Net Carbs: 1g
Sugar: 1g
Fiber: 0g
Fats: 4g
Protein: 2g
Calories: 53

CHAPTER 18

SOUPS & SALADS

Creamy Broccoli Soup

The perfect comfort food, low carb style! This recipe will have you wondering how this could possibly have veggies in it! Super creamy and decadent to hit the spot and pairs perfectly with any main meal.

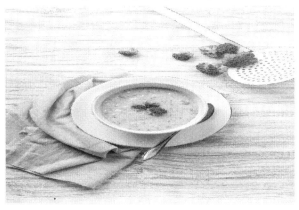

Dietary Label: (GF, EF)
Serves: 4
Prep Time: 10 minutes
Cook Time: 10 minutes

Ingredients:

- 1 head of broccoli, trimmed and chopped
- 3 cups of chicken broth
- 1 cup of heavy cream
- 2 cloves of garlic, chopped

- ¼ cup chopped onion
- 1 cup cubed avocado
- 1 tsp. salt
- ½ tsp. black pepper
- 1 Tbsp. coconut oil

Directions:

1. Start by adding the coconut oil into a large stockpot over medium heat. Add in the onion, and garlic and sauté for 3 minutes. Add in the remaining ingredients minus the avocado and simmer for 5-10 minutes or until the broccoli is tender.

2. Add the avocado into a large food processor or blender, and add to the soup mixture. Blend until super smooth!

3. Enjoy this creamy deliciousness.

Serving Suggestions: Serve with a keto style wrap or alongside any dinner dish.

Substitutions:

- Swap out the avocado if desired, this will just create a less creamy consistency.

Nutritional Information:

Carbohydrates: 17g
Net Carbs: 10g
Sugar: 5g
Fiber: 7g
Fats: 32g
Protein: 7g
Calories: 361

Vegetable Soup

A nourishing veggie soup to bolster the immune system and provide the body with lots of vitamins and minerals. This soup is so yummy you won't even notice how healthy it is!

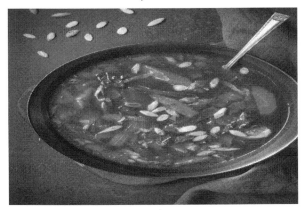

Dietary Label: (GF, EF, DF, V)
Serves: 4
Prep Time: 10 minutes
Cook Time: 10minutes

Ingredients:

- 1 large carrot, chopped
- 1 scallion, chopped
- 1 white onion, finely chopped
- 4 cups of chicken broth
- 1 handful of fresh chopped spinach
- 1 tsp. sea salt
- 1 tsp. black pepper

Directions:

1. This recipe is so easy to make; anyone can throw this together in under 10 minutes! All you need to do is add all of the ingredients into a large stockpot, and bring to a simmer for 10 minutes.

2. That's all there is to it, serve and enjoy!

Serving Suggestions: Serve with a keto style wrap, or enjoy has a nourishing snack.

Substitutions:

- Swap out the spinach for kale if desired.

Nutritional Information:

Carbohydrates: 6g
Net Carbs: 5g
Sugar: 2g
Fiber: 1g
Fats: 1g
Protein: 2g
Calories: 32

Asparagus Bacon Soup

A hearty spin on asparagus soup with a bacon flare! For all, you bacon lovers out there here is a nice way to get in your veggies while still enjoying your bacon. This recipe is super creamy with subtle hints of asparagus.

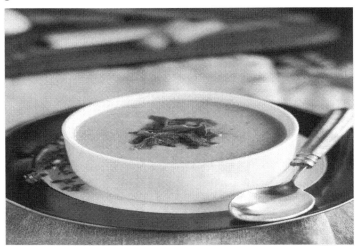

Dietary Label: (GF, EF,)
Serves: 6
Prep Time: 20 minutes
Cook Time: 45 minutes

Ingredients:

- 1 bunch of asparagus
- 4 bacon strips
- ½ of a chopped onion
- 1 Tbsp. coconut oil, melted
- 2 garlic cloves
- 2 cups of chicken broth
- 1 cup of heavy cream
- 1 tsp. sea salt

Directions:

1. To start, preheat the oven to 375 degrees F, and line a baking sheet with parchment paper. Add the asparagus spears and garlic cloves to the sheet and drizzle with the coconut oil. Roast for 12-15 minutes, or until the asparagus is tender.

2. Add all of the ingredients into a stock pot, and simmer for 30-35 minutes.

3. Using an immersion blender, blend until smooth. Season with salt.

4. While the soup is cooking, add the bacon into a skillet and cook until crispy. Crumble once cooked and cooled.

5. Serve the asparagus soup topped with bacon.

Serving Suggestions: Serve with a salad or a keto style wrap.

Substitutions:

- Eliminate the bacon and replace with cheese if desired.

Nutritional Information:

Carbohydrates: 4g
Net Carbs: 3g
Sugar: 2g
Fiber: 1g
Fats: 19g
Protein: 4g
Calories: 195

Fresh Chicken Salad

A light and refreshing salad packed with healthy fats, and protein. This is the perfect complement to any main meal or even serves as an excellent lunch dish.

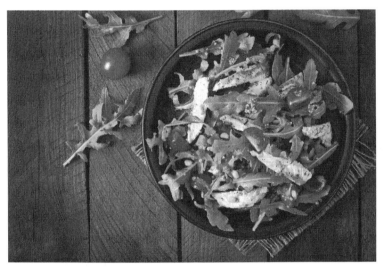

Dietary Label: (GF, EF, DF)
Serves: 2
Prep Time: 10 minutes
Cook Time: 10 minutes

Ingredients:

- 4 cups of arugula
- 8 cherry tomatoes, halved
- 1 chicken breast cut into strips
- 1 tsp. cumin
- ½ tsp red pepper flakes
- 1 Tbsp. olive oil
- 1 Tbsp. freshly squeezed lemon juice
- ½ tsp. black pepper
- 1 Tbsp. coconut oil for cooking

Directions:

1. To start, simply add the coconut oil into a sauté pan over medium heat. Slice the chicken breast into strips, and sauté until cooked through. Season with cumin, and red pepper flakes and cook for another 2-3 minutes.

2. Next, add the greens into a large mixing bowl, and drizzle with the olive oil and the freshly squeezed lemon juice. Top with the halved cherry tomatoes, and sliced chicken breasts.

3. Split into 2 servings, and enjoy!

Serving Suggestions: Serve with soup, or main dish

Substitutions:

*   Swap out the lemon juice for balsamic vinegar if desired.

Nutritional Information:

Carbohydrates: 5g
Net Carbs: 3g
Sugar: 3g
Fiber: 2g
Fats: 16g
Protein: 15g
Calories: 216

Arugula Tomato Salad

Another light salad to accompany a soup or keto friendly wrap. Light and refreshing and low in carbs with a kick from the red pepper flakes.

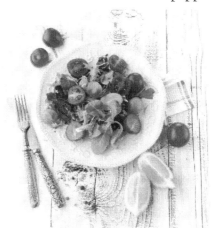

Dietary Label: (GF, EF, DF, V)
Serves: 2
Prep Time: 5 minutes
Cook Time: 0 minutes

Ingredients:

- 4 cups of arugula
- 1 cup of assorted tomatoes, sliced in half
- 2 Tbsp. freshly squeezed lemon juice
- ½ tsp. sea salt
- ¼ tsp. red pepper flakes

Directions:

1. To assemble this simple, refreshing salad, add all of the ingredients minus the lemon juice and seasoning into a large mixing bowl. Toss to combine

2. Drizzle with lemon juice, and season with salt and red pepper flakes,

3. Split into 2 servings and enjoy!

Serving Suggestions: Serve with a bowl of soup or a keto friendly wrap.

Substitutions:

- Swap out the red pepper flakes for a less spicy option.

Nutritional Information:

Carbohydrates: 6g
Net Carbs: 4g
Sugar: 4g
Fiber: 2g
Fats: 0g
Protein: 2g
Calories: 30

CHAPTER 19

DESSERT RECIPES

Coconut Ice Cream Popsicle

You can now have dessert without the guilt while still enjoying all the delicious flavors! These coconut ice cream popsicles are free of refined sugar, creamy and delicious.

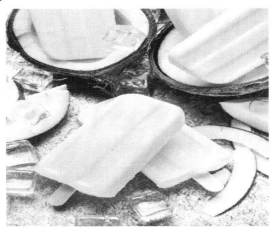

Dietary Label: (GF, EF, DF, V)
Serves: 6
Prep Time: 10 minutes + Chilling time
Cook Time: 0 minutes

Ingredients:

- 2 cups of full-fat coconut milk
- 4 Tbsp. freshly squeezed lemon juice
- ¼ cup shredded coconut

Directions:

1. Simply place all of the ingredients into a blender, and blend until smooth,

2. Transfer into popsicle molds, and freeze for 6 hours or until firm.

3. Enjoy as you would a regular Popsicle!

Serving Suggestions: Serve as a refreshing dessert or even as a guilt-free snack!

Substitutions:

• Swap out the lemon juice for lime juice if desired.

Nutritional Information:

Carbohydrates: 6g
Net Carbs: 4g
Sugar: 3g
Fiber: 2g
Fats: 20g
Protein: 2g
Calories: 198

Nutty Fudge

Who doesn't love a good homemade fudge? Now you can have your fudge and eat it too! Rich and decadent and bake free.

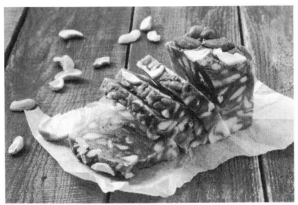

Dietary Label: (GF, EF, DF, V)
Serves: 8
Prep Time: 10 minutes
Cook Time: 5 minutes

Ingredients:

- 1 cup of coconut oil
- ½ cup of peanut butter
- 1 cup of raw cashews
- ¼ cup almonds for topping
- 2 Tbsp. raw cocoa powder
- 1 tsp. pure vanilla extract
- 1 tsp. sea salt

Directions:

1. To make this bake free fudge, add the coconut oil, peanut butter, cocoa powder, vanilla, and sea salt into a saucepan over low heat, and stir until melted. Remove from heat, and add in the raw cashews, stir to combine.

2. Transfer into a parchment lined loaf pan, and top with the almonds.

3. Freeze for 3-4 hours or until firm.

4. Slice and enjoy once hardened, and store leftovers in the freezer.

Serving Suggestions: Serve with a dollop of unsweetened whipped cream for a decadent dessert. (Note this would make this recipe not vegan, or dairy free)

Substitutions:

• Swap out the almonds if desired.

Nutritional Information:

Carbohydrates: 9g
Net Carbs: 7g
Sugar: 1g
Fiber: 2g
Fats: 46g
Protein: 8g
Calories: 454

Hazelnut Avocado Pudding

Finally, a pudding that doesn't come loaded with sugar! This avocado pudding is creamy and resembled that traditional chocolate pudding, so many of us love. This is a fancy pudding naturally flavored with hazelnuts.

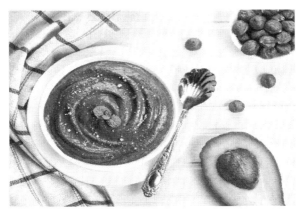

Dietary Label: (GF, EF, DF, V)
Serves: 6
Prep Time: 10 minutes + Chilling time
Cook Time: 0 minutes

Ingredients:

- 4 ripe avocados, pitted and peeled
- ½ cup of unsweetened cocoa powder
- ¼ cup hazelnuts, shell and skin removed
- ½ cup of coconut milk
- 1 tsp. pure vanilla extract

Directions:

1. Simply add all of the ingredients into a food processor, and blend until super smooth.

2. Split among 6 different serving glasses or bowl, and chill for 1-2 hours before serving.

3. Enjoy!

Serving Suggestions: Serve with a dollop of unsweetened whipped cream if desired. (Note this would make this recipe not vegan, or dairy free)

Substitutions:

- Swap out the hazelnuts if desired.

Nutritional Information:

Carbohydrates: 14g
Net Carbs: 5g
Sugar: 0g
Fiber: 9g
Fats: 22g
Protein: 5g
Calories: 245

Matcha Green Tea Chia Pudding

A brand new spin on chia pudding with an even healthier flare! This chia pudding is loaded with antioxidant properties making it the perfect guilt-free dessert.

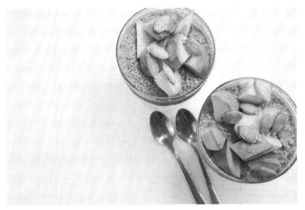

Dietary Label: (GF, EF, DF, V)
Serves: 4
Prep Time: 5 minutes + Chilling time
Cook Time: 0 minutes

Ingredients:

- 1 cup of coconut milk
- ½ cup chia seeds
- ½ tsp. pure vanilla extract
- 1 tsp. matcha green tea powder
- 1 drop of vanilla crème stevia
- 1/2 avocado chopped
- 1 Tbsp. pumpkin seeds

Directions:

1. To make, all you need to do is place the chia seeds, coconut milk, vanilla, stevia, and matcha green tea into a blender, and blend until smooth.

2. Transfer the chia seed mix into a bowl, cover and refrigerate for 4-6 hours or overnight.

3. Split into 4 serving dishes and top with the chopped avocado and pumpkin seeds.

Serving Suggestions: Serve with a dollop of unsweetened whipped cream if desired. (Note this would make this recipe not vegan, or dairy free)

Substitutions:

- Swap out the pumpkin seeds for another nut of choice for topping.

Nutritional Information:

Carbohydrates: 17g
Net Carbs: 5g
Sugar: 2g
Fiber: 12g
Fats: 27g
Protein: 7g
Calories: 317

Raw Brownie

A raw brownie made without flour so you can enjoy a brownie even when living a low carb lifestyle. This recipe is packed full of delicious and nourishing ingredients.

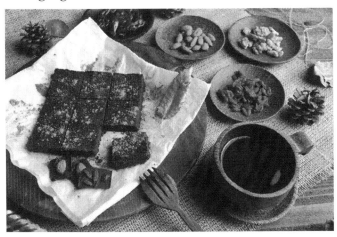

Dietary Label: (GF, EF)
Serves: 16
Prep Time: 15 minutes
Cook Time: 0 minutes

Ingredients:

- 3 cups of raw walnut pieces
- ½ cup of unsweetened cocoa powder
- 4 pitted Medjool dates (Soaked for 20 minutes to soften)
- 2 tsp. pure vanilla extract

Directions:

1. To start, line a large baking sheet with parchment paper.

2. Next, process the walnuts and cocoa powder in a food processor until fine. Add in the soaked pitted Medjool dates. Process until the mixture comes together adding in 1 tsp. of water at a time until the mixture comes together.

3. Flatten the mixture onto the pre-lined baking sheet, and freeze for 4 hours or until hardened.

4. Cut into brownie bars.

Serving Suggestions: Serve with crushed walnuts, goji berries, and almonds if desired. (Note, not reflected in nutritional information)

Substitutions:

- Swap out the pure vanilla extract for peppermint extract for a peppermint flavored brownie.

Nutritional Information:

Carbohydrates: 6g
Net Carbs: 3g
Sugar: 2g
Fiber: 3g
Fats: 15g
Protein: 4g
Calories: 160

CONCLUSION

Thank you so much for reading my ketogenic diet book! I hope that you have found this book resourceful and entertaining and that you are excited as I am to get started on your ketogenic diet. This diet is very simple to partake because it does not require too much work like other fad diets. You now have valuable knowledge to create your own culinary masterpieces in the kitchen that are very healthy, delicious to eat, and physically beautiful to look at. I hope that the recipes have inspired you to get into the kitchen and whip up some delicious, and easy recipes that are low in carbs and high in nutritional value. You will now impress the family at dinner get together and friends who come over for the weekend because you are now the master chef. You have become the "keto" warrior equipped with recipes like a Shaolin master.

I hope these recipes will take you far!

Let's have a brief summary of everything covered in the book:

The great thing about the keto diet is the simplicity in eating the right foods that will contribute positively to your weight loss goals. Moreover, this is an all-natural choice that does not cost too much money, unlike other fad diets, but require more toleration to remove certain foods from your menu to allow the body to fast and get into a ketosis state. You have learned that the ketosis diet is essentially a low carb way of eating to limit the amount of extra energy that the body does not use that eventually get turned into fat. Consuming too much sugar and carbs are some of the main reasons people stay overweight. The keto diet helps to bypass all of this.

The keto diet began in the 1920s and was originally used to treat epilepsy. However, it has really become popular as of late as many people are taking interest in it. Keto dieting was originally used to treat epilepsy in children and have now expanded to a broader range of health benefits.

A person needs to determine whether this diet plan will work for them by factoring in if they take blood pressure or diabetic medication. It is best to consult a qualified healthcare practitioner about any diet plan before putting your life at risk. Your body may or may not be able to handle the pressure.

Achieving ketosis takes time and work and may not show results immediately. Nothing is perfect the first time around unless it is beginner's luck. During ketosis, you need to address how many ketones are in your blood, if the number is high only then is it working. Some ways to measure ketones is by purchasing a personal home meter or setting up a doctor's visit. Ketosis makes you turn into a "fat burning machine" by shedding pounds quickly if done right. This quick weight loss is what has piqued people's interest and made "ketogenic dieting" one of the top Google searches of 2016. Another way of completing a keto diet regimen is by reducing the amount of carbs you consume by adding more good fat to your meals that fill you up more quickly and a bit of protein to top it off.

Completely depriving yourself of life's most precious and pleasurable things, such as eating good food, is never a good idea. However, sticking with the tasty recipes in this book can help you lose weight while enjoying good old fashion food. There are many "keto" friendly healthy foods that will increase your chances of becoming ketogenic, but others will decrease your chances. However, staying organized and creating a reliable meal plan will help you reach health goals faster. Digital apps will help along the journey by logging how many calories, how much protein, carbs and fat you are consuming on a daily basis when you input the information. Documenting your food consumption will help you succeed on the way.

Surprisingly, most people become confused about fats and think they are all bad. Certainly, this is not the case because some are very good to make part of your everyday diet. Targeting the good fats is the best decision you could make because it will actually help you to lose weight. More fat = more weight loss. So, add more good fat to your diet and watch the bad fat shed away! There were many recipes and advice covering how you can comfortably integrate a healthy amount of fat into your diet regimen.

I also talked about the concept of having a "cheat day" where you would indulge in your favorite meal once every 1-2 months just to keep sane during the diet. This cheat day is vital because sticking to the same foods daily becomes kind of boring. This is why it is best to try new foods and mix familiar ones together by using many culinary cooking utensils to create unique dishes.

It is easy to simplify your life with keto dieting because there are many tips in this book that will help you out. Avoiding certain foods, not depriving yourself of certain things, always staying hydrated, getting the right amount of salt (preferably sea salt) into your diet, consuming proteins, electrolytes, good carbs and fasting for a short period just to get your body in the rhythm of ketosis, testing your ketone levels, and doing everything will all help ease the process of ketosis.

Some of the common mistakes made in ketogenic dieting are eating too much carbs. Let's face it, consuming carbs and sugar are addicting and are one of the reasons we eat food in the first place. It is normal for the average person to accidentally consume a large amount of carbs and this is why measuring the exact servings in each fruit and vegetable would serve you well. Some people end up eating too much protein and not enough fats, but luckily we covered the foods that have a good amount of fat and protein.

Moreover, I talked about the idea of staying patient through this whole ordeal because nothing happens overnight. Staying patient would get you in the mindset of staying disciplined to your health goals. You would feel better about all the decisions you make now.

The basis of ketogenic dieting is reducing the amount of sugar and carbs you consume daily. So, it is best to always choose the best alternatives and make better lifestyle choices by eating smaller and more frequent meals as they will help your body achieve optimal health. Avoiding artificial sweeteners and take supplements to get the vitamins and minerals you need is so important in keto dieting, along with getting enough sleep and always exercising because it all helps out tremendously.

I covered 40 mouthwatering recipes that are very healthy and look delicious. This is the meat and potatoes of the book. Now you can cook them and enjoy them.

Involving yourself with a ketogenic dieting is the number one step to achieving a natural state and healthier lifestyle. Many people are getting into the ketogenic diet for various reasons, including losing weight and treatment for epilepsy, among other things. The beautiful aspect about ketogenic dieting is that it is not unnatural, like other diet fads because you choose exactly what to eat. Ketogenic dieting is still somewhat new on the diet scene and was trending for a while. Still, it is one of Google's most popular searches, so people are definitely interested in the way to lose a nice chunk of weight in only ten days. You now have the recipes in your arsenal, along with pictures of how each dish look and the procedure to execute the process. This shows you are in control and can create real masterpieces with only kitchen utensils. Ketogenic dieting may have its side effects, especially in people diagnosed with diabetes, high blood pressure, and those taking medications. Always consult a professional healthcare practitioner to be sure that your diet choice is healthy. Thank you for reading this book and I hope you have gotten some valuable information. Ketogenic dieting for better health!

The ketogenic diet has many perks, and may be the answer for helping assist you in your weight loss goals! Thank you again for taking the time to read my book, and I wish you lots of health and happiness.

Happy keto cooking!

Finally, if you enjoyed this book, then I'd like to ask you for a favor, would you be kind enough to leave an honest review of this book on Amazon? Let others share and experience what you already have. It would help people who are looking for the same information as you to know if this is a book for them or not, and it would be **greatly appreciated!**

Go to bit.ly/KetoBook **to leave a review for this book on Amazon!**

Thank you and good luck!

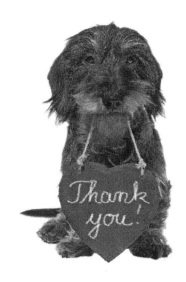

Recipe Index:

Creamy broccoli soup #114
Vegetable soup #117
Asparagus bacon soup #119
Fresh chicken salad #122
Arugula tomato salad #124
Coconut ice cream popsicles #126
Nutty Fudge #128
Hazelnut avocado pudding #130
Matcha green tea chia pudding #132
Raw brownie #134

Made in the USA
Lexington, KY
16 July 2017